W0038445

Clinical and
Ethical Dilemmas
in Palliative and
End-of-Life Care

What Do I Do Now?: Palliative Care

SERIES EDITOR

Margaret L. Campbell, PhD, RN, FPCN
Professor
Wayne University College of Nursing
Detroit, Michigan

VOLUMES IN THE SERIES

Clinical and Ethical Dilemmas in Palliative and End-of-Life Care
Pain
Pediatric Palliative Care
Respiratory Symptoms

Clinical and Ethical Dilemmas in Palliative and End-of-Life Care

Edited by

Daniel B. Carr, MD, FABPM

Professor Emeritus of Public Health and Community Medicine
Program Director and Founder of MS in Pain
Tufts University School of Medicine
Boston, MA, USA

Ann Berger, MD, MSN

Senior Clinical Advisor
Special Volunteer National Institutes of Health Clinical Center
Department Pain and Palliative Care

Adjunct Professor
Georgetown University Medical Center
Division Whole Person Health and Wellness

Adjunct Professor
University of Maryland School of Medicine
Division of Palliative Care

Scientific Advisor
JQ Consulting LLC

Advisor for Sacrospace
Research and Well Being Programs
West Palm Beach, USA

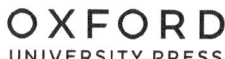

OXFORD
UNIVERSITY PRESS

OXFORD
UNIVERSITY PRESS

Oxford University Press is a department of the University of Oxford.
It furthers the University's objective of excellence in research, scholarship,
and education by publishing worldwide. Oxford is a registered trade mark of
Oxford University Press in the UK and certain other countries.

Published in the United States of America by Oxford University Press
198 Madison Avenue, New York, NY 10016, United States of America.

Library of Congress Cataloging-in-Publication Data
Names: Carr, Daniel B., editor. | Berger, Ann, editor.
Title: Clinical and ethical dilemmas in palliative and end-of-life care /
    Daniel B. Carr MD, FABPM, Ann Berger MD, MSN.
Description: New York, NY : Oxford University Press, [2025] |
    Series: What do I do now?: palliative care | Includes bibliographical references and index.
Identifiers: LCCN 2024049639 | ISBN 9780197681541 (paperback) |
    ISBN 9780197681565 (epub) | ISBN 9780197681558 (ebook) |
    ISBN 9780197681572 (ebook) | ISBN 9780197681589 (ebook)
Subjects: LCSH: Terminal care—Moral and ethical aspects. |
    Palliative treatment—Moral and ethical aspects.
Classification: LCC R726 .C564 2024 | DDC 616.02/9—dc23/eng/20241217
LC record available at https://lccn.loc.gov/2024049639

DOI: 10.1093/med/9780197681541.001.0001

Printed by Integrated Books International, United States of America

Dedicated to my children, Nora, Rebecca, and Andrew, and the memory of my late wife Justine.

—Daniel B. Carr

Dedicated to my husband Carl, my son and his fiancé Stephen and Gabe, and my daughter Rebecca, whose love and support have made my work possible.

—Ann Berger

Contents

Foreword

As we navigate the continuously advancing landscape of health care, we are often confronted with the intricate interplay of medicine, ethics, and the human condition. The chapters in this book reflect our collective journey through some of the most challenging and transformative scenarios in medical practice.

The book opens by exploring family conflicts in information sharing, examining the complex dynamics of familial relationships and the delicate balance between transparency and privacy in patient care. This sets the stage for the subsequent chapters, each offering insightful analyses of the ethical and practical dilemmas encountered at the crossroads of life and death. Chapters such as that on hydration and artificial nutrition at the end of life challenge us to rethink the meaning of sustenance and dignity in our final moments, whereas chapters on selecting comfort care and pediatric intensive care unit cases underscore the diversity of patient needs and the importance of tailored care.

As we delve deeper, the book confronts us with delivering difficult news and tackles controversial medical practices such as physician-assisted death and pain and substance use disorders. These subjects, fraught with differing societal views, present a continuous struggle for families and health care providers as they strive for understanding, empathy, and improved patient outcomes. The book does not shy away from the darker facets of health care—addressing pain, addiction, conflict, and loss in chapters that give a voice to these issues. Yet within these narratives, there is an unwavering quest for compassion and better care.

In the final chapters, readers are prompted to reflect on the wider aspects of health care, such as the mental well-being of providers concerning burnout and resilience, the personal challenges in planning and facing retirement, and the sobering reality of dying alone. Promising insights into innovative patient care approaches, the book concludes with discussions on introducing novel treatments and navigating institutional policies, surrogate decision-making, and approaching palliative sedation at the end of life.

In summary, this book not only guides health care professionals through the multifaceted decisions and circumstances they face but also shines as a beacon of hope that with shared knowledge and experience, we can traverse these waters with heightened empathy and skill. The issues presented within these chapters are a testament to the ever-evolving nature of health care and the enduring spirit of those who dedicate their lives to it.

Salahadin Abdi, MD, PhD

Preface

Health care workers—and certainly oncologists—increasingly practice "personalized" medicine. Paradoxically, this term is now often used to convey the pivotal role that objective, impersonal molecular markers including gene sequencing and receptor typing play in informing diagnosis and treatment. Yet many common clinical and ethical dilemmas confronted on a daily basis in palliative care and supportive oncology reflect family and other relationships gone awry, economic and social strains, clashes of values and beliefs, intergenerational conflict, and other truly personal dynamics. Much of the wisdom that draws junior colleagues to more senior ones to ask "What do I do now?" is based on the latter's ability to sort out complex and changing interpersonal dynamics, reliance on incomplete information, and a high likelihood of emotionally charged conversations erupting into clashes. We are unaware of texts in palliative and supportive care whose primary purpose is to close the gap between the clear, logical, and harmonious clinical world of textbooks and the chaotic, turbulent, resource-constrained, and often unpredictable world of everyday practice. Yet inadequate preparation of trainees to deal effectively with everyday clinical and ethical dilemmas contributes to stress, anxiety, and burnout in young staff. In health care education, the ability to apply practical knowledge in changing circumstances, often with incomplete information, differentiates rote learning of curricula from full clinical competency.

We have assembled a highly respected, interprofessional group of clinicians and health care educators and presented them with clinical vignettes. We asked them to provide concise advice with key points as if to a junior colleague who pulled them aside for a "corridor consult." Most chapters are co-authored by junior and senior colleagues; many address current topics such as the impact of gender identity on care or threats of violence. We hope the reader will use this volume to stimulate discussions among interdisciplinary teams and guide clinicians for whom their training has left them feeling unprepared in confronting everyday dilemmas.

Daniel B. Carr
Ann Berger

Contributors

Salahadin Abdi, MD, PhD
The University of Texas
MD Anderson Cancer Center

Anna Barreiro Albán, BS, MPH, MS
Public Health Consultant

Antje M. Barreveld, MD
Tufts University School of Medicine
Newton-Wellesley Hospital

Ann Berger, MD, MSN
University of Maryland School of Medicine

S. Ian Borison, PhD
Johns Hopkins University School of Medicine

Wesley W. Boyette, MD
OhioHealth Physician Group

Ylisabyth Bradshaw, DO, MS
Tufts University School of Medicine

Mary K. Buss, MD, MPH
Tufts University School of Medicine

Daniel B. Carr, MD, FABPM
Tufts University School of Medicine

Sudha Chandrasekhar, MD, FAAP, MPH, MS
INOVA LJ Murphy Children's Hospital

M. Jennifer Cheng, MD
National Institutes of Health
Clinical Center

Sylvia Christie, MSN, ACNP-BC, ACHPN
Hospital of the University of Pennsylvania

Constance Dahlin, MSN, ANP-BC, ACHPN, FPCN, FAAN
MGB-Salem Hospital
Center to Advance Palliative Care

Shiella Dowlatshahi, MSc
Tufts University School of Medicine

Anthony Eidelman, MD
University of Rochester

Betty R. Ferrell, PhD, MA, CHPN, FAAN, FPCN
City of Hope

Regina M. Fink, PhD, APRN, CHPN, AOCN, FAAN
University of Colorado Anschutz
Medical Center

Carmen Renee Green, MD
City University of New York
School of Medicine

Emily P. Guinee, BS
National Institute of Mental Health

Stephen Gullo, PhD
Institute for Health and Weight
Sciences

Pragya B. Gupta, MD,
FRCS(Edin), DABPM
University of Kentucky College of
Medicine

Beth B. Hogans, MS, MD, PhD
Johns Hopkins University

Marta Illueca, MD, Mdiv, MS,
FAAP
The Yale Program for Medicine,
Spirituality & Religion

Nnamdi C. Iwuala, MBBS
Centra Medical Group

Sharon Kim, DO
National Institutes of Health
Clinical Center

Abigail Lebovitz, MD, MPH
Tufts University School of
Medicine

Angela K. M. Lipshutz,
MD, MPH
National Institutes of Health
Clinical Center

Gabriel Lutz, MD, PhD
University of Maryland School of
Medicine

Steven Mach, MD
The University of Texas
MD Anderson Cancer Center

Margaret M. Mahon, PhD,
CRNP, FAAN, FPCN
National Institutes of Health
Pain & Palliative Care Service

Moe Norton-Westbrook, DNP,
AGPCNP-BC
Memorial Sloan Kettering
Cancer Center

Elizabeth Pasternak, MS, RN,
CHPPN
C.S. Mott Children's Hospital

Carol Pilgrim, NP, FNP-BC
Tufts Medical Center

Justin Price, MD
University of Maryland School of
Medicine

Nafiisah B. M. H. Rajabalee,
MBBS
West Virginia University

Pamela Ressler, MS, RN,
HNB-BC
Tufts University School of
Medicine

Lauren Shaiova, MD
One Brooklyn Health

Deborah J. Snyder, MSW
National Institute of Mental Health

Scott A. Strassels, PharmD, PhD
Wake Forest University School of
Medicine

Baraa O. Tayeb
King Abdulaziz University

Tamara Vesel, MD
Tufts University School of
Medicine

Zhu Wang, MD
Johns Hopkins Hospital

Jennifer Winegarden, DO, MS
Mayo Clinic Health System

PART I

Dilemmas Related to Patients

1 A Choice of Comfort Feeding

Wesley W. Boyette and
M. Jennifer Cheng

A 91-year-old woman with a history of advanced dementia and dysphagia has recently developed increasing difficulty with eating while residing at a nursing home. She was noted to have an increased frequency of coughing spells after meals and progressive weight loss during the past several months. Previously, her diet was adjusted to better manage her dysphagia; however, she continues to have these symptoms. You decide to talk with the patient and her family about this current issue and your concern regarding her declining condition. Based on this discussion, the family and patient agree to enroll her in hospice and focus on her comfort and quality of life. At the end of the conversation, a family member states, "She had always complained about the food she was given after her diet was changed. Now that we are focusing on her comfort, would it be okay to bring her some homemade food that she would enjoy?"

What do you do now?

This case presents a common clinical scenario involving an acute change in condition with worsening dysphagia that necessitates a discussion of nutritional support at the end of life. This discussion is often necessary when a patient has a declining condition or when the patient is unable to take in the necessary amount of nutrition to maintain life. A decision must be made regarding continuing treatment via artificial nutrition with a gastric tube versus forgoing further interventions with artificial nutrition and focusing on comfort. This can understandably be a challenging conversation to navigate, especially with cultural and personal beliefs surrounding nutrition, because the choice is frequently portrayed as withholding food or "starving" a loved one.

One important aspect of having this discussion is verifying that the persons involved in medical decision-making are present or informed of the discussion, especially if the patient lacks the capacity to make complex medical decisions on their own. If the patient maintains capacity, they maintain their autonomy to make decisions regarding their own health; however, at times it may be prudent to have family or persons involved with the patient assist with decision-making so that they are aware of the patient's wishes. This is important because in many cases, a patient may not have the capacity to make a decision on their own, and a surrogate decision-maker or a person designated as health care power of attorney would have to assist with making decisions on the patient's behalf. Regarding the legality of a surrogate decision-maker to make decisions concerning artificial nutrition, the U.S. Supreme Court's decision in *Cruzan v. Director, Missouri Department of Health* supported a patient's right to forgo gastric tube insertion, even when the decision is through a proxy decision-maker.[1] However, despite this court decision and an abundance of literature indicating the lack of benefit in end-of-life situations, discussions regarding continued nutrition remain a common source of distress for families and providers.[1]

WHAT IS COMFORT FEEDING?

In this case, the patient's family mentioned that she had not been enjoying the food she has been eating recently and asked about bringing her food that she can enjoy. This illustrates a good example of the benefit of comfort feeding. Comfort feeding is easiest to describe as a medical order that focuses on providing nutrition for comfort and to minimize patient distress. This can have multiple benefits for the patient and their family because it can expand the patient's diet choices by discontinuing any carbohydrate or sodium restrictions, and monitoring of nutritional status, including tracking meals and calories as well as weighing the patient, may be discontinued.[2] And as this case illustrates, it can give freedom to the family to bring the patient food that they know the patient may enjoy and to share meals together again. Being able to share these benefits can help both providers and families have a better understanding of what the option of discontinuing or forgoing artificial nutrition entails and decrease the discomfort in choosing this focus of care.

In these discussions, being succinct that comfort feeding is the best way to meet patients' needs and provide comfort at this point in their disease process, rather than stating that nutrition is being discontinued, can help avoid misunderstandings regarding care. In addition, providers should be mindful of the cultural and religious considerations of forgoing enteral feeding, including beliefs that food is symbolic of love and caring and that "dying with a full stomach" is important.[3] It can be challenging to talk about nutrition with patients who hold these cultural beliefs, where "starvation and dehydration" may be viewed as cruel ways of dying.

To approach the conversation, it can be helpful to discuss the natural dying process, which includes a gradual reduction in the patient's overall food intake as they continue to decline due to their underlying disease or condition. Loss of appetite and weight loss are normal and expected aspects of the dying process, and explaining this can help bridge understanding for family members concerned about starvation. Regarding enteral feeding, studies demonstrate higher mortality rates in advanced dementia patients with gastric tube placements, as well as no difference in length of survival with or without tube feeding.[4,5] Also, multiple complications can result from gastric tube placement, including leakage, peristomal infection, aspiration, bleeding, and traumatic removal of the catheter.[4,6] A review of patient and family perspectives retrospectively found that at the time of gastric tube placement, patients and families were unaware of common issues of irritation by the gastric tube, use of restraints to prevent traumatic removal of the catheter, use of medications to calm or sedate the patient, and frequent emergency room visits due to complications of the gastric tube.[6] Discussing these complications with patients and their families before a gastric tube is placed enables them to have a better understanding of both tube feeding and comfort feeding and why comfort feeding may be more appropriate.

Comfort feeding should be described in detail. It is typically achieved through careful hand-feeding, which can be adjusted based on clinical conditions to minimize distress or discomfort. Because there is the risk of aspiration, it is important to discuss strategies to reduce this risk with patients and families. This may include recommendations for positioning in bed or in a chair while eating, adjustment of diet with specific textures, reduction in volume per bite, and minimizing distractions during meals. Some recommendations to reduce aspiration may limit the types of food a patient may eat, so carefully weighing the risks and benefits is paramount when developing an individualized care plan with comfort in mind. Freeing the patient from restrictions in diet can be viewed as a form of empowerment for the patient and their family because they can now choose meals for themselves and how to approach nutrition again, promoting quality of life and dignity of the patient. Reviewing these factors enables patients and families to make informed decisions regarding the best care for the patients.

> Following a thorough discussion with the family, a shared decision
> was made to adjust the patient's diet to focus on comfort feeding.
> After a few weeks, you receive a report that the patient is now un-
> responsive and has not attempted to eat for the past several days.
> The family requests guidance on how to best address her needs, in-
> cluding her nutrition.

In this case, it is appropriate to stop feeding because the patient is nearing the end of life. The focus of comfort feeding should always be the patient's comfort and align with their clinical condition to maximize comfort and minimize harm. If feeding is causing distress, it is appropriate to respect the patient's wishes and avoid causing undue harm. Allow the patient to take the lead through this process. Often, this can be accomplished by periodic re-evaluation of the patient and, if the patient's alertness is fluctuating, offering food when they are able to easily take in the food for comfort. In addition, some patients may have the sensation of thirst and dry mouth may develop as they continue to decline, and can be well managed even when they can no longer swallow liquids with good oral hygiene and oral lubrication.[7]

Ongoing communication between the health care team and the family is important to provide continued psychosocial-spiritual support and alleviate symptoms that their loved one may experience as they go through the normal dying process. The patient in this case exhibits signs of further decline and short prognosis, so continued feeding is likely not feasible and could cause distress. Understandably, this can be a difficult time for families as they process changes in the patient's condition. Being available to assuage their worries and educate them on expected end-of-life symptoms and signs can improve understanding and acceptance of the current care goal.

KEY POINTS TO REMEMBER

- Comfort feeding is a medical order that focuses on providing nutrition for comfort and to minimize patient distress.
- Be mindful of family or cultural considerations in regard to nutrition. Describing comfort feeding and the natural dying process can help alleviate stress for the patient and family.
- Frequently, patients will need continued re-evaluation and reinforcement regarding nutrition at the end of life, and maintaining communication is paramount to ensure comfort for patients and their families.

References

1. Palecek EJ, Teno JM, Casarett DJ, Hanson LC, Rhodes RL, Mitchell SL. Comfort feeding only: A proposal to bring clarity to decision-making regarding difficulty with eating for persons with advanced dementia. *J Am Geriatr Soc.* 2010;58(3):580–584. https://doi.org/10.1111/j.1532-5415.2010.02740.x
2. Orrevall Y. Nutritional support at the end of life. *Nutrition.* 2015;31(4):615–616. https://doi.org/10.1016/j.nut.2014.12.004
3. Ngan OMY, Bergstresser SM, Sanip S, Emdadul Haque ATM, Chan HYL, Au DKS. Cultural considerations in forgoing enteral feeding: A comparison between the Hong Kong Chinese, North American, and Malaysian Islamic patients with advanced dementia at the end-of-life. *Dev World Bioeth.* 2019;20(2):105–114. https://doi.org/10.1111/dewb.12239

4. Blomberg J, Lagergren J, Martin L, Mattsson F, Lagergren P. Complications after percutaneous endoscopic gastrostomy in a prospective study. *Scand J Gastroenterol.* 2012;47(6):737–742. https://doi.org/10.3109/00365521.2012.654404

5. Lee Y-F, Hsu T-W, Liang C-S, et al. The efficacy and safety of tube feeding in advanced dementia patients: A systemic review and meta-analysis study. *J Am Medical Directors Assoc.* 2021;22(2):357–363. https://doi.org/10.1016/j.jamda.2020.06.035

6. Teno JM, Mitchell SL, Kuo SK, et al. Decision-making and outcomes of feeding tube insertion: A five-state study. *J Am Geriatr Soc.* 2011;59(5):881–886. https://doi.org/10.1111/j.1532-5415.2011.03385.x

7. Hammond L, Chakraborty A, Thorpe C, O'Loughlin M, Allcroft P, Phelan C. Relieving perception of thirst and xerostomia in patients with palliative and end-of-life care needs: A rapid review. *J Pain Symptom Manage.* 2023;66(1):e45–e68. https://doi.org/10.1016/j.jpainsymman.2023.02.315

2 Patients Seeking Alternative Treatments for Cancer Pain

Steven Mach and Salahadin Abdi

Tony, a 35-year-old male, presents to your clinic with the chief complaint of abdominal pain. He has a recent diagnosis of stage II pancreatic cancer, which was found incidentally on health screening for life insurance. Computerized axial tomography showed a mass in the pancreatic head with local spread to nearby lymph nodes. The patient is otherwise healthy and has not needed any prior health maintenance. His abdominal pain is getting progressively more debilitating and prevents him from getting sleep at night or going to work. He describes his pain as a vague dull ache that is localized to his epigastric area. The patient works as a firefighter and notices that his pain worsens with movement such as climbing stairs. He says that he does not like taking medications, although he has recently tried acetaminophen and ibuprofen with minimal relief. He reports that he lives a "natural lifestyle" and consumes mostly "plant-based products." Currently, the patient is open to starting chemotherapy as directed by his oncologist, although he is specifically inquiring about nontraditional medicines and alternative therapies for his cancer pain.

What do you do now?

As the health care provider for this patient, it is important for you to assess the patient's values and goals for treatment. The patient is determined to trial nontraditional therapies for cancer pain and is asking for your guidance. Although numerous alternative treatments are available, many are yet to be supported by research-driven or evidence-based medicine. At the core of providing a pain management plan, especially if the patient is seeking care outside of medical purview, is patient safety.

Alternative medicine (AM) gradually become popular in recent decades, especially among cancer patients. The terms *complementary* and *alternative* refer to products or practices that are not part of the conventional treatments offered by licensed medical professionals. Although these terms are often used interchangeably, there is a clear difference between the two modalities: Complementary therapies are used *alongside* traditional treatments, whereas alternative therapies are nonconventional methods used *instead of* standard medical care. "Integrative" care may combine various elements of AM with a focus on the interplay between biologically based systems such as botanical supplements, nutrition, exercise, mental health, mind–body practices, and spirituality.

The patient, Tony, returns to your clinic and reports that he started chemotherapy but has experienced gastrointestinal issues and is now considering stopping his cancer treatment and starting an "herbal remedy" that his friend mentioned. You recall that a 2020 survey by the American Society of Clinical Oncology reported that 35% of Americans believe that cancer can be cured by alternative therapies alone.[1] Although some non-mainstream approaches to treating oncologic symptoms have gained traction, there is little or no scientific evidence proving the efficacy of AM to cure cancer. In addition, one study found that among cancer patients who used AM therapies, 29% did not tell their doctors.[2] The conventional stepwise approach to cancer pain management often involves an array of pharmacologic agents ranging from acetaminophen to nonsteroidal anti-inflammatory drugs, opioids, and adjuncts (e.g., antidepressants, anticonvulsants, and corticosteroids). Fittingly, it is essential that a practitioner works closely with a patient who is thinking about using AM because many deleterious drug–drug interactions exist between AM and conventional medications. As described below, replacing standard of care with alternative treatments can be dangerous or even life-threatening.

Clear, specific indications for AM are frequently lacking and require continued research. There is no substantial evidence to support the use of AM for cancer pain in published trials due to small sample sizes, heterogeneity of study design, and high risk of study bias.[3] Currently, much of what is known about AM is anecdotal and patient-reported. From a provider standpoint, a reasonable goal is to openly discuss nontraditional therapies as an adjunct that may improve pain and quality of life (e.g., stress, anxiety, depression, nausea, and sleep) but not to replace or negatively interact with other therapies with proven effectiveness for cancer pain (i.e., opioids, surgery, chemotherapy, or radiation).

On follow-up, Tony reports that he now has extreme fatigue from the chemotherapy. He asks if there are any techniques or exercises that you recommend. From your experience with similar patients, you recollect that there are some common complementary therapies that some patients self-report, which are less likely to cause harm or interfere with conventional treatments for cancer pain.[4] Acupuncture, based in traditional Chinese medicine, involves stimulating points on the body to potentially help with mild pain and some nausea; biofeedback uses monitoring devices to help patients learn how to control normally automated physiologic functions such as heart rate, blood pressure, and muscle tension; massage therapy can help relieve pain, stress, anxiety, depression; yoga and tai chi both combine movement with controlled breathing to help relax the body/mind and improve strength/balance; reiki is based on the concept that energy flows throughout the body and uses hands placed around the body to guide that energy for healing purposes; spirituality and prayer can help some patients manage the emotional component of cancer pain; art or music therapy can enhance mental wellness and improve quality of life; and guided imagery may help focus positive images in the mind such as scenes or experiences to relieve stress and pain. As with many ailments, optimizing physical health through exercise/movement and a well-balanced diet is recommended. Such complementary techniques are intended to help patients manage pain and symptoms while they undergo standard cancer pain treatments provided by a medical doctor.

A few weeks later, Tony has another health maintenance appointment and reports that he is starting to have painful burning and numbness in his hands and feet from the chemotherapy. In addition to his cancer treatment, he is starting to take a mixture of "healing herbs" that he purchased at a local apothecary. You advise Tony that AM strays away from evidence-based medicine in its use of vitamins, dietary supplements, or botanicals. It is important to emphasize that just because these products claim to be "natural" does not mean they are always safe to consume. The AM herbal supplements can have toxic side effects or negatively interact with other medications or cancer treatments. Even when the product is consumed as intended, many have side effects such as hypertension, hepatotoxicity, and neurologic sequalae/symptoms.[5] Most of these products can be bought "over the counter" and are not regulated by the U.S. Food and Drug Administration. Moreover, AM products are limited by quality control; there is an inconsistency in biologic potency, product sourcing, and contamination prevention, thus detracting from the reliability of many AM products.

Numerous botanical supplements contain chemically active compounds, which can interfere with pain medications, chemotherapy, biologics, and other medical management. Specifically, many chemotherapy drugs are metabolized in the liver by the cytochrome P450 isotypes, a group of enzymes commonly affected by numerous botanical and herbal remedies.[5] For example, St. John's wort, commonly used for depression, is an inducer of CYP3A4, which can increase the breakdown (and therefore decrease the efficacy) of oxycodone as well as chemotherapeutic regimens such as taxanes, irinotecan, and imatinib. Conversely, essiac, commonly promoted as an anticancer herbal tea, can inhibit CYP3A or act as an immunosuppressant to potentiate the effects of cytotoxicity. Another commonly consumed AM is green tea, which contains polyphenols that can both inhibit and induce several P450 enzymes. Other prevalent inducers of the CYP enzymes include panax ginseng (for alertness) and gingko biloba (for memory), which also increase the metabolism of chemotherapeutic agents. On the other hand, plants such as milk thistle, promoted as a dietary supplement for liver function, have been shown to decrease the metabolism of cancer drugs such as paclitaxel and doxorubicin. Furthermore, herbs such as berberine, although sold as anti-tumor products, can reduce the vulnerability of cancer cells to cytotoxic agents. When discussing AM use, it is essential for the provider to have a candid and open conversation about vitamins, supplements, and herbals and advise patients about the potential interactions that these botanical agents have on conventional pain medications and chemotherapeutics. After discussing the possible side effects of AM with Tony, he decides to consider all his options and will come back to clinic.

Aside from the intrinsic toxicities of AM medications, there is additional risk of delaying or avoiding well-established treatments for cancer and pain. Although there are sparse studies on the direct harms of refusing standard medical care, research indicates that patients who pursue alternative therapies instead of conventional cancer therapy tend to be younger, female, of higher socioeconomic status/education level, and live in the western United States. Those who chose AM, compared to patients who received only conventional cancer treatments, had higher rates of refusal of surgery, radiation therapy, chemotherapy, and hormone therapy. Alternative therapy was also associated with a lower 5-year survival rate and greater mortality risk, likely mediated by delay or refusal of conventional cancer care.[6] Although the existing research is purely observational, it suggests that alternative therapies need not replace nor hinder standard medical treatment.

For many patients enduring the challenges of cancer pain, AM can serve as an outlet for personal empowerment. Patients may feel like they are participating in their own care when they add their personalized regimen or self-medicate, sometimes with the belief that these alternate methods can eliminate cancer pain or cure cancer. Nonetheless, for a health care provider, there is a fine line between guidance and deterrence of AM. By openly discussing the patient's wishes without judgment or rejection, the provider can strengthen patient rapport.

As proponents for patient safety, it is prudent for providers to talk about AM with an objective perspective. Although AM is not rigorously studied, that does not necessarily mean it has no potential benefit for cancer pain, nor preclude it from future investigation. However, if a patient is determined to replace their conventional care with AM, advocating for caution is appropriate. AM treatments that claim to "end cancer pain," "cure cancer," have "no side effects," are "miracle/secret/breakthrough" therapies, or instruct patients to avoid standard medical treatment should be inspected with wariness. Although a provider cannot stop a patient from seeking alternate therapies, it behooves both parties to question treatments with no proven scientific evidence. Providers should highlight the lack of evidence for AM with impartiality, not necessarily to refute it but, rather, to seek more extensive research from trustworthy sources to fill in gaps of knowledge.

On returning for follow-up, Tony reports that he decided to continue his chemotherapy and will pause on taking any over-the-counter herbal supplements for his cancer pain. He appreciates that you listened to his point of view and are advocating for his well-being. Your approach continues to focus on an unbiased conversation with the patient about their treatment goals and values. Judiciously guiding the patient to complete their course of chemotherapy before starting any alternative therapies results in the patient receiving verified conventional medical treatment and avoids any potentially unpredictable medication interactions. All the while, the proven benefits of complementary therapies, such as mindfulness and exercise, can be leveraged to improve cancer pain and quality of life alongside standard of care.

KEY POINTS TO REMEMBER

- There is a lack of evidence to prove that alternative therapies are effective in replacing standard medical treatments for cancer pain.
- Many cancer patients seek alternative medicine for their cancer treatment without informing their physicians.
- It is important to have open and unbiased conversations with patients about alternative therapies, highlighting safety concerns and need for further safety and efficacy research.
- Many vitamins/supplements/herbs can negatively interact with or reduce the efficacy of treatment for cancer pain or chemotherapy.
- Encourage patients to not replace or avoid standard medical treatments for cancer pain.
- Activities with a high benefit to risk potential, such as acupuncture, biofeedback, yoga, tai chi, spirituality, art/music therapy, balanced diet, and exercise, can help improve quality of life.

References

1. American Society of Clinical Oncology. *Cancer Opinions Survey*. American Society of Clinical Oncology; 2020.

2. Sanford NN, Sher DJ, Ahn C, Aizer AA, Mahal BA. Prevalence and nondisclosure of complementary and alternative medicine use in patients with cancer and cancer survivors in the United States. *JAMA Oncol.* 2019;5(5):735–737.

3. Bao Y, Kong X, Yang L, et al. Complementary and alternative medicine for cancer pain: An overview of systematic reviews. *Evid Based Complement Alternat Med.* 2014;2014:170396.

4. American Cancer Society. The truth about alternative medical treatments. n.d. https://www.cancer.org/latest-news/the-truth-about-alternative-medical-treatments.html

5. Grigorian A, O'Brien CB. Hepatotoxicity secondary to chemotherapy. *J Clin Transl Hepatol.* 2014;2(2):95–102. doi:10.14218/JCTH.2014.00011

6. Johnson SB, Park HS, Gross CP, Yu JB. Complementary medicine, refusal of conventional cancer therapy, and survival among patients with curable cancers. *JAMA Oncol.* 2018;4(10):1375–1381.

Delivering Difficult News as a Covering Provider

S. Ian Borison

Mrs. R is a 65-year-old dental hygienist who presented with dyspnea for the past week, as well as epigastric pain for months. Her pain was not responding to the over-the-counter nonsteroidal anti-inflammatory drugs she had been taking. During her evaluation, she was found to have significant microcytic anemia, leading to admission for workup of symptomatic anemia. She was found to have melenic stool, and gastroenterology was consulted. An esophagogastroduodenoscopy was performed showing two gastric ulcers, which were clipped and biopsied.

You are the oncoming hospitalist starting your shift on Saturday morning and you receive a call from the gastroenterologist. They tell you that the preliminary pathology shows gastric adenocarcinoma, but molecular and genetic testing will take a few more weeks to return. The patient has not yet been notified of the results. Because they will not be back until Monday, the gastroenterologist requests your help in breaking the news to the patient.

What do you do now?

DISCUSSION

Delivering difficult news is a stressful part of being a health care provider, and it can be more anxiety-provoking when there have been few or no opportunities to build a relationship with the patient. Focusing some of your time on building a rapid rapport can help ease the experience and allow for a smoother interaction. Employing a stepwise approach to these conversations can help reduce stress for you and the patient.[1]

Before seeing the patient, it is important to prepare for delivering difficult news. Anticipate questions the patient or their loved ones may ask about this new diagnosis, such as "What can be done in terms of treatments?" Consider discussing the results and treatment plans with any relevant consultants so that you are properly prepared to answer questions that may arise (while understanding that some of these questions will need to be deferred to specialists or until further information is available). Consider discussing with the gastroenterologist which specialists should be consulted, such as oncology and general surgery. This is an appropriate time to discuss the case with oncology to ensure proper workup is initiated. Ask if there are imaging studies that should be ordered for staging or other workup the oncologist would order for the eventual consultation visit. After preparing a reasonable amount of information to answer any relevant questions about what comes next, set aside an appropriate amount of time to meet with the patient and discuss the difficult news. Identify an appropriate setting for discussing the information, such as a quiet and private patient room or family meeting room.

When first meeting the patient, spend time building reasonable but rapid rapport. Start with the basics. Make eye contact and introduce yourself and your role to the patient. Begin the encounter with a general evaluation prior to discussing the news, which will build rapport by showing your concern regarding their symptoms and well-being. Practice active listening and show genuine interest in the patient. Ask the patient to tell you a bit about themself to start to get to know them on a personal level. These are underappreciated and often overlooked steps for building a rapid relationship with a patient.

After completing your necessary initial evaluation and building some rapport, transition the conversation to a discussion surrounding the patient's preferences regarding information sharing. You can normalize this by stating there are certain questions you ask all patients to better understand their values. Ask how the patient likes to be informed of updates about their health care. Do they prefer to hear updates alone, or do they have loved ones they would like present for any discussions? Information preferences can also include the level of detail the patient prefers. Some patients prefer to hear every detail about their test results, diagnosis, prognosis, and treatment plans. Other patients prefer a big picture approach, focusing on the provider's impression and how this applies to the patient's clinical situation. Understanding the patient's preferences for information sharing will allow you to tailor your delivery to meet their needs. Although this will not change the content of the difficult news, it can help give the patient a sense of control while providing the information in its most easily digestible form.

After evaluating the patient's information-sharing preferences, honor these wishes. If they have loved ones they would like present, arrange for a meeting with them. A popular mnemonic device for a stepwise approach to delivering difficult news is SPIKES: *s*et-up, *p*erception, *i*nvitation, *k*nowledge, *e*mpathy (responding to emotions), *s*trategy (and/or next steps).[1] The first step is the set-up, which includes the process outlined above as well as choosing an appropriate location for the meeting. Ensure an appropriate amount of time is set aside and that there is a private meeting space with minimal distractions.[2]

Prior to discussing the news, it is important to first understand the patient's perception of their condition and if they have any anticipation of the coming news. Address the fact that you and the patient are starting a new relationship and reassure them that you have reviewed their medical history. Ask the patient what information their health care team has shared with them and what they understand about their condition. Consider stating something like "I have reviewed your chart and I see that there has been a lot happening since you have been in the hospital. I wonder what you have heard from your doctors?" Assessing the patient's understanding will help determine where to start with your information sharing.

After assessing the patient's understanding of their disease, ask permission to share the new information that you have obtained. This step is called invitation in the SPIKES mnemonic. This is not only polite and courteous but also gives the patient the opportunity to let you know their preferences for receiving information if they choose.

Prior to meeting with the patient to deliver the difficult news, develop a succinct and meaning-based sentence to convey the news. It is important to include the information, as well as an explanation of the meaning behind that information. After the patient gives permission to share information, consider a warning shot before delivering the news. For instance, you may state, "The biopsy results have returned and unfortunately, I have unexpected news; it shows that you have stomach cancer. This means we will need to do more testing and discuss treatment plans." After delivering this news, the patient will need some time to process the information. Allow for a silent moment. Resist the urge to fill the silence with more information, and provide the patient an opportunity to process and respond.

Expect an emotional response after sharing difficult news and be prepared to respond with empathy. After receiving difficult news, patients will often respond with questions that seem cognitive; however, they are likely driven by strong emotions. For instance, a statement such as "Are you sure this is cancer? Couldn't it be something else?" is likely more heavily emotional than cognitive and therefore requires an emotional response. Responding to emotional questions with cognitive answers will not address the underlying concern of the patient and will not allow the discussion to progress. When a person is having an emotional response, it is difficult to process information and think clearly. Therefore, the focus should be on addressing the emotional response before addressing information that requires cognitive processing.

There are many techniques for addressing emotions that can be helpful in these situations; however, the most important aspect is to ensure the responses are genuine and empathic. A helpful mnemonic for responding to emotions is NURSE: *n*aming, *u*nderstanding, *r*espect, *s*upport, *e*xplore.[3]

Naming is a technique in which the clinician acknowledges emotions the patient is displaying. This gives validity to the emotions and allows the patient an opportunity to address their response to the news. It is important to be suggestive of the emotions, rather than declarative, because this is an imperfect science and meant to allow the patient to express their feelings, which generally deescalates emotional responses.[3]

Expressing understanding is a helpful technique, such as responding with "This news must be so difficult to hear." Avoid statements that imply you understand exactly what the patient is experiencing, such as "I know what this is like, and you will get through this." This statement prematurely provides reassurance and is more likely to be inflammatory than soothing.

Respect and support are other patient-centric ways of addressing emotions. Respect can be conveyed by acknowledging the patient's efforts, such as their ability to advocate for themselves and endure long and difficult treatments, or acknowledging their coping mechanisms when hearing difficult news. Reinforcing your support of the patient can be in the form of reassuring them that no matter the outcomes of testing or treatment, you will be there to help guide and support them. These reassurances are commonly overlooked therapeutic devices the provider has available to them.

The last technique of the NURSE mnemonic is to explore. This can be done by asking the patient about the emotions or thoughts they are experiencing in order to help you address their specific concerns. It can also be an invitation to patients to explore their own emotions and reactions to help them process. Using these techniques can help address the emotions that patients experience when receiving difficult news and lower the emotional temperature to allow for next steps to be discussed.

After addressing the emotions and answering any questions, the next step is to strategize, which means to discuss the path forward in the context of the news. If there are multiple different paths forward, this is an opportune time to complete a values assessment to help guide recommendations for next steps. Using a transitional statement can allow the discussion to shift toward planning for the future. Consider asking about the patient's biggest hopes and worries in the context of the news. This can help guide your recommendations for the next step. When providing recommendations, frame them in the context of the values the patient shared and describe how that information helped you formulate your recommendations.

CASE RESOLUTION

When asked about information preferences, Mrs. R shares that her sister is a nurse and therefore Mrs. R would like her sister and her spouse to be present when new information is shared. The patient's loved ones come to visit the hospital in the early afternoon for a meeting. The meeting takes place in the patient's private hospital room, and the SPIKES mnemonic is used as guidance for the meeting. The biopsy results are shared in clear and simple terms, and the patient and family are in disbelief and quite upset at first. The clinician is able to respond to their emotions using the NURSE mnemonic, and the emotional temperature is significantly reduced. Next steps are discussed, including plans for an oncology consultation and computed tomography (CT) scans of the chest, abdomen, and pelvis.

The results of the CT scan show some gastric wall thickening but, more important, no evidence of lymphadenopathy or distant metastatic disease. General surgery is consulted with a plan for outpatient follow-up in 1 week for surgical planning of a partial gastrectomy. The patient is discharged home with her family with prescriptions for her gastric ulcers and appointments with the general surgery and oncology clinics.

KEY POINTS TO REMEMBER

- When there is a need to discuss difficult news with a new patient, focus on building rapid rapport and determining the patient's preferences with regard to receiving medical information.
- Deliver the news in a patient-centered, stepwise approach, with guidance from the SPIKES mnemonic.
- Deliver the news in a concise and meaning-based sentence, preceded by a warning shot.
- After delivering the news, expect an emotional response, and respond to emotional questions with empathy using the NURSE mnemonic.
- After responding with empathy, consider completing a values assessment and discussing next steps with the patient.

References
1. Baile WF, Buckman R, Lenzi R, Beale EA, Kudelka AP. SPIKES—A six-step protocol for delivering bad news: Application to the patient with cancer. *Oncologist.* 2000;5(4):302–311.
2. Berkey FJ, Wiedemer JP, Withalani ND. Delivering bad or life-altering news. *Am Fam Physician.* 2018;98(2):99–104.

3. Back AL, Arnold RM, Baile WF, Tulsky JA, Fryer-Edwards K. Approaching difficult communication tasks in oncology. *CA Cancer J Clin*. 2005;55(3):164–177.

Additional Resources

Helpful online tools and guides to these conversations can be found on the Ariadne Labs website: https://www.ariadnelabs.org/serious-illness-care/for-clinicians.

For courses focused on discussing and delivering serious news, visit the VitalTalk website: https://www.vitaltalk.org.

4 To Pray or Not to Pray: Is That the Question?

Marta Illueca

Your patient is asking you to pray with them. Family members attend a local church and regularly pray amongst themselves. You have different religious beliefs and feel uncomfortable. Your beliefs are at odds with their beliefs, and the hospital chaplain is on leave. Your patient, who has been cared for by you for many years, has expressed a high degree of fondness and rapport towards you. Rather than have you be just a simple and passive observer, your patient is pleading for you to be a willing and active participant of their devotional practice. They also want the health care team on duty to spend a few minutes together in prayer at the beginning of a shift or at least on morning rounds. Some of the nurses are on board because spiritual care is a mandatory aspect of their bedside training, and they are sensitive to the devotional needs of patients. This request is starting to strain the health care team's collaborative spirit.

What do you do now?

DISCUSSION

Can Praying Be Therapeutic Rather Than a Coping Strategy in Sickness?

In order to answer this question, we need to start by explaining what exactly is prayer. An extensive discussion of the meaning of prayer is beyond the scope of this chapter; however, let us seek some common ground to aid in understanding the suggested approach to this clinical case.

Simply stated, prayer is an ancient practice of peoples throughout the world in an effort to honor a higher power and procure a grace or a benefit on their own behalf (e.g., healing, plentiful crops, good fortune, longevity, etc.). The *Oxford Dictionary of English Etymology* indicates that the word "prayer" derives from the Old French *preier*, meaning "to request," and it originated in the 13th century from the Medieval Latin noun *precarious* (i.e., *entreaty*) and the verb *precare*, which means "to ask earnestly, beg, entreat."

The global and widespread growth of religions and the many forms of spiritual communing with a higher power have confounded the original meaning of "prayer." In current times, health care practitioners, scientists, and academic researchers tend to conflate various types of devotional practices under the same umbrella, including, but not limited to, meditation, mantra chanting, and the various types of prayers (e.g., praise, thanksgiving, lamentation, contrition, contemplation, centering, etc.).

Because of the evolution of the prayer practice into a multidimensional concept,[1] the wholistic definition of prayer as cataloged by *Encyclopedia Britannica* is used in this chapter. Prayer is defined as "an act of [personal] communication by humans with the sacred or holy—God, the gods, the transcendent realm, or supernatural powers." Of note, a person need not be religious in order to pray, and praying may be practiced by anyone who is open to the idea of requesting help from a transpersonal source of benevolence, real or imagined. In this regard, prayer indeed could be conceived as therapeutic if it makes the patient feel better physically, mentally, and/or spiritually. The empirical basis of this proposition is discussed in the next section.

Do the Prayer Content, Mode of Implementation, and Person's Belief Affect Health Outcomes?

There is a knowledge gap pertaining to the area of the spiritual aspects of patient care. Current literature highlights the limited but substantive empirical data related to the potential benefits of praying by patients with different types of medical conditions, particularly those associated with physical pain.[2,3] The latter includes acute, post-surgical, procedural, and chronic (including cancer and non-cancer) pain. And coupled with the advancement of research on the intersection of spirituality and health, novel and validated psychometric measures are now available to help characterize the spirituality, religiosity, and devotional practices of pain patients. Examples of these are the Duke University Religion Index (DUREL)[4] and the Pain-related PRAYER Scale (PPRAYERS).[5]

The health care team's approach for a patient request for prayer should be assessed with a respectful and open-minded attitude. In this respect, there is a growing body of research data, both qualitative and quantitative, highlighting the potential benefits of certain types of personal prayer, both as a coping strategy and as a potential therapeutic adjuvant within the continuum of complementary and integrative medicine. In the United States, the National Institutes of Health have a dedicated National Center for Complementary and Integrative Health whose mission is "to define, through rigorous scientific investigation, the usefulness and safety of complementary and integrative interventions and their roles in improving health and health care." The time has come, then, to critically review and update the medical fund of knowledge that so far has been the terrain of a purely "biomedical model" but that is gradually shifting toward a "biopsychosocial–spiritual" model.

Highlights of a recent systematic review on prayer and pain[2] indicate that the types of pain-related prayer with more substantive data overall pointed to personal prayer (by the person or with the person who has pain), directed to God or a higher power (versus a secular entity—non-persona) and with a petitionary character. This prayer profile was more statistically significant in terms of pain-related outcomes. From a research standpoint, it is notable that distant intercessory prayer and group-based prayer studies have fallen into disfavor due to methodology challenges and mixed results.

Three thematic domains that were identified in the medical literature which characterize the overall anatomy and physiology of prayer as observed in the setting of pain management are the prayer type (i.e., target and content), the patient profile (i.e., adults, religious or nonreligious), and the clinical scenario (i.e., acute versus chronic pain). The best available literature is supportive of religious prayer directed to God or a higher power (as opposed to a secular entity), with an active "self-motivating" content. All the latter aspects apply specifically to personal prayer in situ as opposed to distant, group-based community prayer that is nonparticipatory on the side of the patient or health care team.

Is There a Patient Profile That Is "Amenable" for Using Prayer as Part of Their Healing Journey?

In the case presented in this chapter, the patient's request, although not unusual, brings a distinctive character to the doctor–patient dichotomy. There may be people whose notion of the universal is nonsectarian. The latter group may include agnostics, atheists, naturalists, and those self-designated as spiritual but not religious. In this case, both doctor and patient are religious but in different denominational arenas. This situation should not preclude finding a strategy to support the patient's spiritual needs while respecting the doctor's religious tenets.

The case illustrates various dichotomies that conform the greater question of "To pray or not to pray?" with our patients. These dyads include the doctor's versus the patient's beliefs, the medical versus the nursing training approaches, and the individual's spirituality or religious backgrounds. With certain thoughtful guidelines, this question can be approached in a sensible and responsible manner. Notably, the nursing literature offers valuable insight into the integration of the spiritual needs of a patient into their day-to-day care (see Further Reading). As it pertains to this specific request for their doctor to pray with them, it is always possible to "pray in parallel."

The description of a "prayer-primed patient"[2] (Figure 4.1) tells us that an adult patient requesting prayer from their health care providers is particularly amenable to the beneficial coping and healing effects of their favored devotional practice, and patients with painful medical conditions are even more open to an integrative team approach for their care. It behooves us as physicians to update ourselves on the emerging literature that highlights

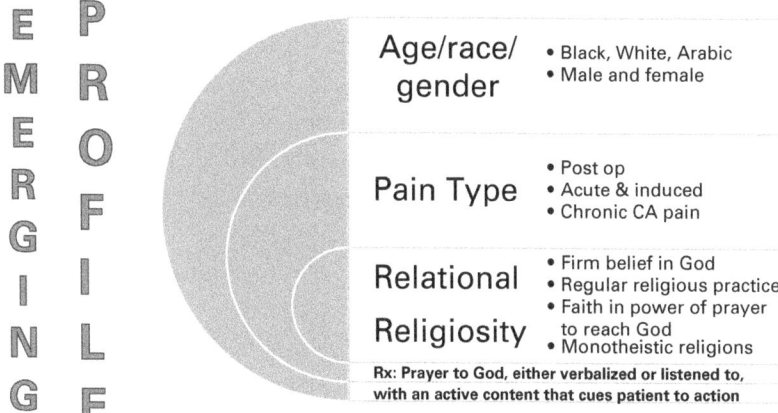

E M E R G I N G	P R O F I L E		

		Age/race/ gender	• Black, White, Arabic • Male and female
		Pain Type	• Post op • Acute & induced • Chronic CA pain
		Relational Religiosity	• Firm belief in God • Regular religious practice • Faith in power of prayer to reach God • Monotheistic religions

Rx: Prayer to God, either verbalized or listened to, with an active content that cues patient to action

FIGURE 4.1 The prayer-primed patient. Based on published data, the prayer-primed patient usually has a monotheistic belief in God and the power of prayer and participates in religious practices. The literature is inclusive of any gender or ethnicity. Studies have included patients with postoperative pain, acute or induced pain, chronic cancer pain, and noncancer pain.[2]

the potential health benefits of prayer for certain types of patients (i.e., believers), both by honoring requests, as in this case, and by preserving the ethics and integrity of the physician and health team members.

CASE RESOLUTION

In this clinical situation, there are more than one potential avenues for resolution. First, if both patient and doctor share a common belief in a higher power, regardless of their individual religions, then they could pray in parallel, letting the patient or a team member lead with a brief prayer. Second, if the doctor decides not to pray due to their different religion, they can offer their patient a silent prayer on their behalf asking for healing according to the tenets of their religiosity. Third, if the doctor rejects the patient's petition, the doctor could still offer their support by enlisting an alternative team member of the same religion as the patient or who is willing to say a brief prayer that is nondenominational and honors the dignity and spirituality of the patient.

There is no set rule for excluding ourselves from a participatory prayer experience that may uplift and console a patient who needs it. In the absence of a chaplain, finding someone from the health care team who shares the same religious background may be a feasible strategic bridge. The person seeking prayer, or a next of kin, may guide those at the bedside and indicate a favorite scriptural or traditional prayer. The prayer "script" can be provided by a family member or the patient. Bedside prayers are typically short, focus on gratitude for a grace received, and solicit healing from a higher power.

KEY POINTS TO REMEMBER

- Because prayer is touted in the medical literature as a pain coping strategy and potentially an adjunct to pain management, it behooves the health care practitioner to allow for this devotional practice to be part of a patient's care plan when such a patient specifically requests so.
- Honoring the patient's own spirituality does not diminish the credibility of the health care team; rather, it increases the rapport and sense of validation for a given patient.
- The provider's own religiosity or spirituality is a crucial part of the patient care equation and must be managed in a comparable sensitive and respectful way.
- Find the common ground. Different religions are colored by both overlapping and contrasting beliefs. Almost all religions acknowledge a belief in a higher power. Many have their own sacred texts or books of prayer. A chaplaincy consult will help sort out a harmonious interfaith approach.

References
1. Puchalski C, Ferrell B, Virani R, et al. Improving the quality of spiritual care as a dimension of palliative care: The report of the Consensus Conference. *J Palliat Med.* 2009;12(10):885–904. https://doi.org/10.1089/jpm.2009.0142
2. Illueca M, Doolittle BR. The use of prayer in the management of pain: A systematic review. *J Relig Health.* 2020;59(2):681–699. doi:10.1007/s10943-019-00967-8
3. Jarego M, Ferreira-Valente A, Queiroz-Garcia I, et al. "Are prayer-based interventions effective pain management options? A systematic review and

meta-analysis of randomized controlled trials. *J Relig Health*. 2023;62(3):1780–1809. https://doi.org/10.1007/s10943-022-01709-z

4. Koenig HG, Büssing A. The Duke University Religion Index (DUREL): A five-item measure for use in epidemiological studies. *Religions*. 2010;1(1):78–85. https://doi.org/10.3390/rel1010078

5. Meints S, Illueca M, Miller MM, Osaji D, Doolittle BR. The Pain and PRAYER Scale (PPRAYERS): Development and validation of a scale to measure pain-related prayer. *Pain Med*. 2023;24(7):862–871.

Further Reading

Beauregard M, Paquette V. Neural correlates of a mystical experience in Carmelite nuns. *Neurosci Lett*. 2006;405(3):186–190. https://doi.org/10.1016/j.neulet.2006.06.060

Breslin MJ, Lewis, CA. Theoretical models of the nature of prayer and health: A review. *Mental Health Religion Culture*. 2008;11(1):9–21, https://doi.org/10.1080/13674670701491449

Büssing A. Measures of spirituality/religiosity—Description of concepts and validation of instruments. *Religions*. 2017;8(1):11. https://doi.org/10.3390/rel8010011

Elmholdt EM, Skewes J, Dietz M, et al. Reduced pain sensation and reduced BOLD signal in parietofrontal networks during religious prayer. *Front Hum Neurosci*. 2017;11:337. https://doi.org/10.3389/fnhum.2017.00337

Koenig HG. *Religion and Mental Health: Research and Clinical Applications*. Academic Press; 2018.

Minton ME, Isaacson M, Banik D. Prayer and the Registered Nurse (PRN): Nurses' reports of ease and dis-ease with patient-initiated prayer request. *J Adv Nurs*. 2016;72(9):2185–2195. https://doi.org/10.1111/jan.12990

Pain and Substance Use Disorder

Baraa O. Tayeb and Antje M. Barreveld

During your morning rounds, you see a 42-year-old female patient with an acute-on-chronic flare of pain from breast cancer surgery and treatment. The patient is complaining of severe, diffuse pain despite being hospitalized for 2 days. She has struggled with pain from a complicated breast reconstruction surgery as well as neuropathic pain from chemotherapy. She has been using alcohol and cocaine to cope with her pain and was admitted for pain control and treatment after a fall while intoxicated. She lives alone.

When you visit her hospital room, she is tearful and in agony. She is thinking of leaving the hospital against medical advice because her pain is not being taken seriously. "No one wants to help me because they think I'm in addict. I can't handle this anymore." When you ask your house staff about the reason for not appropriately escalating her opioids to manage her pain, you are told, "She has a history of substance abuse. Her urine toxicology was positive for cocaine. We don't think opioids are a good idea."

What do you do now?

DISCUSSION

Substance use disorder (SUD) is a disease defined by an overpowering desire to obtain and use substances despite the negative social, professional, and health consequences. SUD does not discriminate by race, ethnicity, gender, or socioeconomic status. Many patients with SUD also suffer from chronic pain. Multiple barriers to evidence-based SUD care (e.g., shame, societal and medical bias and stigma, and inadequate access to evidence-based SUD services) contribute to a long delay between onset of SUD and access to treatment. Acute and chronic pain management in patients with active SUD or in recovery can be particularly challenging, with additional barriers to pain care. Access to pain management without discrimination is a right of every patient. The Psychotropic Substances Act, an amendment to the Controlled Substances Act, prohibits restrictions on opioid prescribing for pain relief. However, indications for opioid therapy should be carefully assessed, and opioids should be prescribed with appropriate safety measures in place to prevent misuse or overdose. A team-based and individualized approach to maximizing pain relief, SUD treatment, as well as safety is essential.

Every pain management plan should start with proper clinical assessment. This includes obtaining a thorough history about the onset and cause of pain, functional impairments, medical history, social and psychiatric history, family history, and physical exam. In addition, a substance use risk assessment can be helpful to identify patients at risk for opioid misuse or relapse. Screening, brief intervention, and referral for treatment (SBIRT) can provide a framework for caring for your patient with active SUD. Validated screening tools identify patients who may need additional support and monitoring. Screening for addiction can be as simple as using a one-question validated questionnaire, such as the National Institute on Drug Abuse (NIDA) Quick Screen, and if positive, a more detailed questionnaire such as the 10-item NIDA Drug Abuse Screening Test (DAST-10) provides additional risk assessment on the severity of the SUD. The Opioid Risk Tool (ORT) delineates risk factors for opioid misuse when starting a new opioid prescription and includes an assessment of the most important risk factors for developing opioid use disorder (OUD): family history of SUD, personal history of untreated psychiatric illness, and personal history of SUD. For patients prescribed opioids, various assessment tools can monitor for risks of opioid misuse, such as the Current Opioid Misuse Measure (COMM), Screener and Opioid Assessment for Patients with Pain–Revised (SOAPP-R), and the Patient Medication Questionnaire (PMQ).

If a patient such as the one in the case presented in this chapter screens positive for SUD, unbiased communication of our concern and options for treatment can help pave the way for recovery. For our patient with an acute flare of chronic cancer pain and cocaine use disorder, the team must weigh the risks and balances of opioid treatment. However, most important, undertreated pain can lead to severe sequelae, including death. Treating cancer pain is essential, and opioids are almost always needed to accomplish this. In our patient with multiple risk factors for opioid-related morbidity and mortality, a patient-centric plan coordinated between the patient and teams, as well as appropriate counseling and monitoring, can ensure safety.

Ideally, our patient will pursue more specialized addiction care, and opioids may be tapered prior to discharge from the hospital as pain improves. Often, however, high doses of opioids are needed to control pain from boney metastases, and they may need to be continued in the outpatient setting. Although our patient may not have a diagnosis of OUD, the patient may benefit from a trial of one of the two U.S. Food and Drug Administration (FDA)-approved opioid medications for OUD that can also be helpful in managing pain: buprenorphine (with decreased risk for misuse and respiratory depression compared with morphine and other pure μ-opioid agonists, this medication can be prescribed in any outpatient setting by anyone with a Drug Enforcement Agency license—special training is no longer required) or methadone (with a long half-life, methadone is dispensed daily by specialized outpatient treatment programs to ensure safety). Counterintuitively, lowering of opioid dose and/or rotation from one opioid to another may sometimes improve pain control, raising the diagnosis of opioid-induced hyperalgesia.

A summary of best practices in managing pain with opioids in our patient with SUD is provided in Box 5.1. If opioids are needed outpatient in our high-risk patient to prevent additional health risks from undertreated cancer pain, a stepwise and harm-reduction approach can ensure safety. Maximizing non-opioid alternatives is paramount and summarized in Box 5.2.

BOX 5.1   **Steps for Opioid Management and Pain Care Planning for the Patient with SUD**

For active SUD, refer for treatment; consider initiating medications for SUD or OUD.
Consult the prescription drug monitoring program to assess for prescribed controlled substances.
Obtain a urine drug screen and monitor routinely (e.g., q2–4 weeks) to help inform care (a positive screen does not mean opioids are contraindicated).
Involve the patient, support network, and interdisciplinary team in the care planning; provide informed consent on the risks of opioids.
Identify an outpatient prescriber and formulate a treatment agreement.
Regularly assess pain intensity and function with frequent in-person visits (e.g., weekly and at least monthly), and screen for opioid-induced hyperalgesia.
Prescribe naloxone (Narcan), and instruct family members/friends in its use.
Regularly assess the "4 A's" (analgesia, activity, adverse effects, and aberrant behaviors).
Periodically review pain as well as substance use; discuss possible taper plans and additional referral to treatment or more intensive outpatient or inpatient SUD treatment if tolerance/OIH suspected.
Document best practices in opioid prescribing and monitoring.

OIH, opioid-induced hyperalgesia; OUD, opioid use disorder; SUD, substance use disorder.

BOX 5.2   **Non-Opioid Pain Management Options**

Multimodal medications (NSAIDs, acetaminophen, muscle relaxants, neuropathic medications, topical analgesics)
Nonpharmacologic treatment (physical therapy, exercise, massage, heat/ice, yoga, chiropractic care, and acupuncture)
Interventional pain management (steroid and local anesthetics injections)
Mind–body and behavioral medicine support (cognitive–behavioral therapy, biofeedback, relaxation strategies, etc.)
Support groups
Distraction aligned with personal interests
Nutritional and anti-inflammatory strategies

NSAIDs, nonsteroidal anti-inflammatory drugs.

CASE RESOLUTION

You completed a full assessment for the patient and conveyed your concern regarding her cocaine use. She was started on low-dose intravenous nonsteroidal anti-inflammatory drugs (ketorolac, caution taken given risks of renal, cardiac, and gastrointestinal toxicity), acetaminophen, and sublingual buprenorphine three times per day for opioid therapy for possible discharge planning and outpatient opioid management. The patient was provided with education concerning opioid tolerance/hyperalgesia, and a low-dose intravenous ketamine infusion was started. After 48 hours, the patient demonstrated marked improvement and the ketamine was stopped. Her primary care physician was contacted to coordinate outpatient buprenorphine prescribing and monitoring, a possible taper plan if indicated as her pain needs evolve. She was provided with intranasal naloxone for safety in case of overdose if illicit substances are used. She was discharged home to follow up with her primary care physician and pain management clinic. She agreed to meet with an addiction specialist for ongoing care, peer, and behavioral support, and an intake appointment was scheduled.

KEY POINTS TO REMEMBER

- Access to pain management without discrimination is a patient right. Care for your patient without bias and without stigma.
- Utilize SBIRT as a framework for supporting your patient with pain and addiction to access appropriate SUD care.
- When indicated, managing pain with opioids in the patient with a history of SUD and potential tolerance/hyperalgesia can be done safely with safety parameters, counseling, and monitoring in place.
- Consider harm-reduction strategies to prevent opioid overdose (e.g., naloxone co-prescribing, utilizing FDA-approved medications for OUD when appropriate, and continuing opioids even when active SUD in certain disease states such as cancer with painful metastases).

• Maximize non-opioid pain management strategies for all patients.

Further Reading

1. Barreveld AM, Mendelson A, Deiling B, Armstrong CA, Viscusi ER, Kohan LR. Caring for our patients with opioid use disorder in the perioperative period: A guide for the anesthesiologist. *Anesth Analg*. 2023 Sep 1;137(3):488–507. PMID: 37590794.

2. Duggirala R, Khushalani S, Palmer T, Brandt N, Desai A. Screening for and management of opioid use disorder in older adults in primary care. *Clin Geriatr Med*. 2022;38(1):23–38. doi:10.4088/pcc.v04n0402

3. Strang J, Volkow ND, Degenhardt L, et al. Opioid use disorder. *Nat Rev Dis Primers*. 2020;6(1):3.

4. Horner G, Daddona J, Burke DJ, Cullinane J, Skeer M, Wurcel AG. "You're kind of at war with yourself as a nurse": Perspectives of inpatient nurses on treating people who present with a comorbid opioid use disorder. *PLoS One*. 2019;14(10):e0224335.

5. Cheetham A, Picco L, Barnett A, Lubman DI, Nielsen S. The impact of stigma on people with opioid use disorder, opioid treatment, and policy. *Subst Abuse Rehabil*. 2022;13:1–12.

6. Wakefield EO, Belamkar V, Litt MD, Puhl RM, Zempsky WT. "There's nothing wrong with you": Pain-related stigma in adolescents with chronic pain. *J Pediatr Psychol*. 2022;47(4):456–468.

7. Moberg DP, Paltzer J. Clinical recognition of substance use disorders in Medicaid primary care associated with universal screening, brief intervention and referral to treatment (SBIRT). *J Stud Alcohol Drugs*. 2021;82(6):700–709.

6 Patient with a Low Respiratory Rate Receiving Opioids

Baraa O. Tayeb and Antje M. Barreveld

You receive a call from the nurse in the hospice residence asking for you to attend to Ms. Smith, who has advanced stage 4 hepatocellular carcinoma. One hour ago, she received 10 mg of intravenous hydromorphone and still is moaning from pain. Her vital signs are as follows: blood pressure 80/44 mmHg, heart rate 50 beats per minute, and respiratory rate six breaths per minute. Her breathing is slow, irregular, and with occasional gasping. She is noncommunicative but appears in pain. Her eyes and mucosa are jaundiced. You believe the patient is still in intractable pain and are considering another dose of hydromorphone, but you and the nurse are concerned about her low respiratory rate.

What do you do now?

DISCUSSION

It is estimated that 25% of dying patients in the last weeks of life have unrelieved pain despite receiving prescribed opioids. Managing pain with opioids at the end of life is an ethical and legal imperative; however, multiple barriers to pain relief exist. For instance, organizations and health care workers may lack the proper protocols, palliative care consultative services, and pain education to adequately manage pain in the terminally ill patient. Additional barriers to managing pain have been identified by health professionals; a fear of hastening death is the most common barrier identified (Box 6.1). From a patient's perspective, additional considerations may contribute to decreased pain treatment at the end of life (Box 6.2). Identifying these barriers and addressing them head-on are the first steps to improving pain care at the end of life.

BOX 6.1 **Health Care Provider Barriers to Adequate Pain Management at the End of Life**

Patient deterioration (e.g., death and addiction)
Concern for legal and professional licensing actions
Lack of knowledge, training, or experience in pain management
Ethical and legal misconceptions
Personal, cultural, and religious beliefs
Patient and/or family willingness to accept personal, cultural, and religious beliefs
Challenges in team, patient, and family communication
Institutional barriers (e.g., adequate staffing, medication availability, pain and palliative care consultancy services, and lack of pain care guidance or protocols)

BOX 6.2 **Patient Barriers to Adequate Pain Management at the End of Life**

Personal, cultural, and religious beliefs
Fear of analgesics side effects, addiction, or death
Knowledge gaps about pain management
Neglect by health care institutions and/or workers

Most important, evidence in the field of palliative care medicine demonstrates that opioids do not hasten a patient's death, even when used for terminal weaning of mechanical ventilation or treatment of agonal breathing. Pain care at the end of life can be summarized by the following principles and best practices:

1. Palliative intent: When opioids are used in palliative care, they are administered with the intent to relieve suffering and manage pain, not to cause or hasten death. Medical professionals may follow established guidelines and protocols to ensure the safe and appropriate use of opioids in end-of-life care.

2. Ethical and legal considerations: In many countries, the law and ethical principles support the use of medications, including opioids, to relieve pain and suffering, even if there is a possibility that these medications may have inadvertent side effects. This is the principle of "double effect," which allows for pain relief even if there are foreseeable but unintended consequences.

3. Patient autonomy: It is essential to engage in open and honest communication with the patient (if possible) and their family, respecting the patient's wishes and goals for care. Decisions about pain management should be made collaboratively, taking into account the patient's values, beliefs, and preferences.

4. Regular assessment: Health care providers should regularly assess the patient's pain and adjust the pain management plan as needed. This may involve titrating opioid doses up or down based on the patient's response and comfort level.

5. Informed consent: Patients and their families should be informed about the potential benefits and risks of pain management options, including opioids. Informed consent ensures that everyone understands the treatment plan and its implications.

6. Multidisciplinary approach: End-of-life care often involves a team of health care professionals, including physicians, nurses, social workers, and chaplains, who work together to provide holistic care and support for both the patient and their family.

In summary, the fear of hastening a patient's death should not be a reason to limit opioid-related pain control at the end of life. Appropriate pain management is a fundamental aspect of compassionate end-of-life care, and health care providers should strive to balance the relief of suffering with the respect for a patient's autonomy and values. Open communication, informed decision-making, and a palliative care approach are essential tenets of pain care at the end of life.

CASE RESOLUTION

After full assessment, you determine the patient should receive an additional dose of hydromorphone. You communicate with the patient's family about adequate pain relief and address the nurse's fear that additional opioid could hasten death. Your patient receives the additional hydromorphone and is resting comfortably. The patient dies within a few days, and the family is appreciative of your care.

KEY POINTS TO REMEMBER

- Twenty-five percent of patients at the end of life have unrelieved pain.
- Recognize that the various health care–related and patient-related barriers to adequate pain care, such as a fear of hastening death, can unnecessarily worsen suffering.
- The principle of double effect applies during pain management for patients at the end of life, allowing for pain relief even if there are foreseeable but unintended consequences.
- There is no evidence that appropriately administered opioids for pain hasten death at the end of life.

Further Reading
1. Klint Å, Bondesson E, Rasmussen BH, Fürst CJ, Schelin MEC. Dying with unrelieved pain: Prescription of opioids is not enough. *J Pain Symptom Manage.* 2019;58(5):784–791.
2. Elmstedt S, Mogensen H, Hallmans DE, Tavelin B, Lundström S, Lindskog M. Cancer patients hospitalised in the last week of life risk insufficient care quality: A population-based study from the Swedish Register of Palliative Care. *Acta Oncol.* 2019;58(4):432–438.

3. Andersson S, Sandgren A. Organizational readiness to implement the Serious Illness Care Program in hospital settings in Sweden. *BMC Health Serv Res.* 2022;22(1):539. doi:10.1186/s12913-022-07923-5

4. Moody K, Baig M, Carullo V. Alleviating terminal pediatric cancer pain. *Children.* 2021;8(3):239.

5. Orujlu S, Hassankhani H, Rahmani A, Sanaat Z, Dadashzadeh A, Allahbakhshian A. Barriers to cancer pain management from the perspective of patients: A qualitative study. *Nurs Open.* 2022;9(1):541–549.

6. Queensland University of Technology. Legal protection for providing pain and symptom relief. n.d. Accessed June 11, 2023. https://end-of-life.qut.edu.au/pain-relief

7. Faris H, Dewar B, Dyason C, et al. Goods, causes and intentions: Problems with applying the doctrine of double effect to palliative sedation. *BMC Med Ethics.* 2021;22(1):141.

8. Coyle S, Elverson J, Harlow T, et al. The myth that shames us all. *Lancet.* 2018;392(10154):1196.

9. UpToDate. Ethical considerations in effective pain management at the end of life. n.d. Accessed October 11, 2023. https://www.uptodate.com/contents/ethical-considerations-in-effective-pain-management-at-the-end-of-life#:~:text=Pain%20management%20at%20the%20end%20of%20life%20is%20the%20right,in%20the%20United%20States%22

Video Gaming and Virtual Reality in Pediatrics

Elizabeth Pasternak and Pamela Ressler

Jake, who recently turned seven during his hospitalization for a stem cell transplant, has shown significant withdrawal from both his family and healthcare providers. He spends most of his time immersed in video games, isolating himself and avoiding meaningful interaction. This behavior has been particularly challenging for his family, who feel powerless and uncertain about how to connect with him in a supportive way.

In addition to his social withdrawal, Jake has exhibited behaviors that pose risks to his medical care. He has attempted to pull out his peripherally inserted central catheter (PICC) line when he thinks no one is watching, raising serious safety concerns for the health care team. While they want to address Jake's behavior, they are unsure of how to approach the issue without placing blame or causing further distress.

The health care team hopes that the unit child life specialist can provide strategies to help Jake express his emotions and process his hospital experience. Given Jake's strong engagement with video games, they are exploring the possibility of using them in a more structured way to help reduce his anxiety and discomfort.

What do you do now?

DISCUSSION

Undergoing a stem cell or bone marrow transplant can be a difficult and stressful experience for individuals of any age, especially so for school-age children. Currently, stem cell transplantation involves prolonged hospitalizations and protective precautions, including physical isolation for many, to prevent infection during the post-transplant period.

Proactive early involvement of child life specialists to work with adaptive coping strategies and developmental skills can be important for a school-age child such as Jake. Therapeutic play is crucial to social, emotional, and cognitive development and is even more critical during adversity or stress points in a child's life, such as a stem cell transplant. Establishing a trusting relationship with health care professionals can also assist in addressing fears and anxiety associated with displacement from peers and familiar routines.

Jake's frequent use of video games may be helpful during his treatment and recovery. Jake seems to find familiarity and comfort in playing video games, and as such they can be used to enhance his hospital environment. It is important to validate that many school-age children and adolescents dealing with a serious illness engage in video games, virtual reality (VR), and augmented reality as tools to improve the hospital experience and healing process. Such activities may allow Jake the opportunity to maintain relationships with peers and establish new connections despite being confined within a hospital room, creating a bond of normalcy with nonhospitalized peers or contributing to a feeling of achievement. Video gaming and VR can provide hospitalized children with access to a digital playground in addition to other benefits, including the following:

- Stimulation of fine motor movement, problem-solving, and critical thinking
- Cooperative game play to encourage socialization and normalization
- Reduction in isolation from friends and family outside the hospital through online gaming

CASE RESOLUTION

Jake and his parents meet with the child life specialist on the unit where Jake will be spending his hospitalization. The child life specialist understands that Jake likes to "escape" into the worlds of his favorite video games. After learning a bit more about what types of games Jake likes, the specialist talks about her role and how she can help customize an approach to integrate technology and entertainment into Jake's care plan. She takes the time to talk about the importance of nonpharmacologic therapies and other supportive services that will be available throughout Jake's hospitalization.

The child life specialist also suggests a few new video games that Jake may like to try from the game library in the hospital. She asks Jake and his parents if Jake would like to meet some other kids online who also play the same video games. The child life specialist validates that being sick and hospitalized can often mean a long absence from school that makes kids feel socially isolated. She encourages Jake's parents to help Jake stay connected with classmates and friends at home with the use of social networking sites, email, video messages, and perhaps online video games. In addition, she introduces the concept of a school liaison (school intervention specialist) who can help work alongside Jake and his family to serve as the bridge between the medical setting and the school community.

Exploring coping methods for this hospitalization is essential for Jake to properly adjust to an extended hospital stay. Some school-age children are able to express their worries verbally, whereas others demonstrate their concerns through behavioral changes. Studies have revealed that medical interventions themselves have the potential to be traumatic for patients and families. For a child, a traumatic event can occur when they feel very frightened, out of control, and perceive there is a threat of serious harm or even death to themself or someone else. These experiences can initiate strong emotions and physical reactions that can persist far beyond the traumatic event. Unfortunately, in a hospital setting, there is a high prevalence and significant concern for recurrent exposure to trauma.

Could Jake's perceived lack of control in the hospital setting be the cause of his increasing attempts to dislodge his PICC line?

The health care team meets with Jake and his parents to discuss how Jake has been doing throughout this process. In their experience, school-age children often want to participate in discussions about their care but would rather not bear full responsibility for decision-making. For Jake, it might be about taking part, voicing his preferences, being listened to, and being heard in decisions that ultimately impact his life.

It is important to allow space for Jake and his parents to ask questions and for the health care team to acknowledge the recent event without passing judgment or placing blame. Ideally, this question-and-answer process will allow Jake and his parents to gain an understanding of and responsiveness to the behavior. The question-and-answer process should emphasize continuity of care and collaboration across the health care system.

If Jake is willing, explore what about the PICC line is concerning or bothersome to him. How might a history of trauma have contributed to Jake's acute presentation? Strategize if aspects of Jake's care can be performed differently or more collaboratively. Provide Jake with choices about his care, such as dressing change or medication times, whenever possible, but maintain clear expectations to create opportunities for him to rebuild a sense of control and empowerment. Attempt to identify if Jake has established a therapeutic relationship with anyone on his care team. If not, emphasize the importance of establishing a trusting relationship between Jake and his health care team as a top priority. Consider consulting pediatric psychology and palliative care to provide comprehensive evaluation and treatment recommendations should Jake continue to demonstrate such behavior or develop post-transplant complications that emerge during a longer hospitalization.

KEY POINTS TO REMEMBER

- Child life therapy focuses on the emotional, social, and developmental needs of children, helping patients and their families cope with being in the hospital through play, education, and creative activities. Early referral can help address psychosocial concerns in addition to promote adaptive coping strategies for children living with a serious illness.
- Pediatric illness and injury are among the most common potential emotionally traumatic experiences for children and their families. The application of a trauma-informed approach to medical care has the potential to mitigate these negative consequences.

- Hospitals are using video games, VR, and augmented reality to help encourage socializing, create a distraction, and even aid in therapy. These platforms have the potential to enhance the patient experience and transform the hospital environment.
- An illness can make children feel different and lonely. Connection to peers is important to school-age children, especially during prolonged hospitalizations. School liaisons (hospital school programs) can help bridge between the medical setting and the school community.
- Medical isolation has a significant impact on health, contributing to increased symptoms of depression and anxiety, as well as feelings of fear, abandonment, loneliness, and stigmatization. Lack of control due to medical procedures and hospitalization may lead to regression, emotional withdrawal, or aggressive behaviors such as attempting to dislodge PICC lines or other medical equipment.
- Children who are undergoing or have undergone the process of stem cell transplants face changes in their daily living, including impacts of their diagnosis, symptom burden, aggressive treatments, continuous procedures, and likely post-procedure complications. Early integration of palliative care has been proven to improve patient outcomes.

Further Reading
1. Burns-Nader S, Hernandez-Reif M. Facilitating play for hospitalized children through child life services. *Children's Health Care*. 2016;45:1–21. doi:10.1080/02739615.2014.948161
2. Coyne, I. Children should be more involved in healthcare decisions that affect them. The Conversation. Accessed April 19, 2017. https://theconversation.com/children-should-be-more-involved-in-healthcare-decisions-that-affect-them-74228
3. Delvecchio E, Salcuni S, Lis A, Germani A, Di Riso D. Hospitalized children: Anxiety, coping strategies, and pretend play. *Front. Public Health*. 2019;7:250. doi:10.3389/fpubh.2019.00250
4. For kids in the hospital, video games are part of recovery. *Wired*. Accessed July 2022. https://www.wired.com/story/kids-video-games-gaming-specialists-pediatrics-childs-play

5. Koukourikos K, Tzeha L, Pantelidou P, Tsaloglidou A. The importance of play during hospitalization of children. *Mater Sociomed*. 2015;27:438–441. doi:10.5455/msm.2015.27.438-441

6. Marsac ML, Kassam-Adams N, Hildenbrand AK, et al. Implementing a trauma-informed approach in pediatric health care networks. *JAMA Pediatr*. 2016;170(1):70–77. https://doi.org/10.1001/jamapediatrics.2015.2206

7. Romito B, Jewell J, Jackson M, et al. Child life services. *Pediatrics*. 2021;147(1):e2020040261. https://doi.org/10.1542/peds.2020-040261

8. C. S. Mott Children's Hospital, University of Michigan Health. Therapeutic gaming and digital technology. n.d. https://www.mottchildren.org/mott-support-services/cfl-therapeutic-gaming-and-digital-technology

9. McMahan L. Video games support young patients' social, emotional health. Oregon Health & Science University. Accessed November 23, 2022. https://news.ohsu.edu/2022/11/23/video-games-support-young-patients-social-emotional-health

8   Native American Spirituality and Healing

Marta Illueca

Ted has been admitted to the palliative care unit with an advanced illness. He wants you to hang dreamcatchers at the head of his bed. In addition, he wants you to organize a bedside healing ceremony involving tribal elders like himself, in which they chant prayers, smudge, and prepare a psychedelic herb tea that they all sip together. He insists that his outlook and prognosis under the palliative care team will be more bearable this way. His family is also requesting a large room to accommodate members of his community who want to partake of this ceremony. You do not think the risk-to-benefit assessment justifies any of these requests.

What do you do now?

This case underscores a growing trend in the health care spheres—that of conjoining both conventional and complementary disciplines in a collaborative fashion, namely in an integrative health care model. In this approach, the patient is treated with multidisciplinary approaches and within the continuum of self, community, and environment.

In dealing with Ted's specific requests, it is necessary to balance an empathetic attitude with a scientific understanding of the effects of social isolation and disconnection from what the patient considers a sacred part of their own spiritual essence. Recent scientific literature reports that social and physical pain are registered in the brain through common pathways.[1] In addition, spiritual pain may result from a severance, real or imagined, of a person's connection with the sacred, a circumstance that results in a painful alienation and inability to commune with their own spiritual sense of a higher power.[2] Ted's requests must therefore be pondered within the possibilities of spiritual pain and existential distress.

Keeping the previous discussion in mind, this case requires a general level of understanding of the traditional medicine and healing (TMH) system that is at the core of Native American lifestyle and cultural heritage in North America. An extensive exposition of the philosophical and theoretical tenets of TMH is beyond the scope of this chapter, and the reader is referred to the Further Reading section for an in-depth review. Suffice to say that TMH has been recognized by the National Institutes of Health with the creation in 2015 of the Tribal Health Research Office, which focuses on implementing health-related policies and programs for tribal groups. This case is an excellent example of how an integrative approach to the care of the Native American patient is not only feasible but also mandatory, especially as it pertains to the understanding of its philosophical tenets for wellness, health, and wisdom.

The TMH system is practiced through a multidimensional continuum, including individual, communal, and transgenerational layers. Its theoretical framework is essentially transpersonal and interwoven through a conceptualization of humans as tripartite beings (i.e., formed in body, mind, and spirit). This simple principle is central to the proper and responsible management of Native American patients who crave and demand a health care system that honors their customs and their traditions.

Although there are hundreds of tribal groups, there are certain common themes in their healing systems. There are three key areas representative of their spirituality as it applies to Ted's case.

TMH healing formulas generally consist of the presence of an elder (also known as the "medicine man/woman"), a communal practice (i.e., prayer, smudging, or herbal remedies), and use of a symbolic object (e.g., dream-catcher). It is important to note that TMH interventions are not practices set apart from but, rather, inherent to the day-to-day life of Native Americans. They rely heavily on a lifestyle aimed at maintaining harmony with the created world, the earth's environment, the community, and the universe at large. So in essence, there is nothing in this clinical case that is alien to the profile of a contemporary member of a Native American tribal group.

Although an exhaustive list of practices is beyond the scope of this chapter, it is important to understand a set of principles surrounding the wellness and healing philosophies of Native Americans. The latter constitute a holistic way of life that underpins the requests from Ted and his family. His requested interventions are cardinal components of their wellness practices, and only a minute representation of a much wider wellness and healing armamentarium that has been part and parcel of Native American populations since their origins in North America.

Three key components of their traditional healing system are recognized in Ted's case: a healer/practitioner, a set of spiritual practices, and the use of special objects.

THE PRACTITIONER—THE HEALER—THE ELDER—THE MEDICINE MAN

The requested practitioner is an elder who is to facilitate the healing ceremony and communal gathering. The bedside ceremony is the most basic spiritual practice that lies at the core of the Native American philosophy of life, which recognizes a creator entity, a created earth/universe, and a created self. It is believed that through prayer, spoken or chanted, the individual may commune with the creative energies of the universe and its creator, and thus find healing and wholeness. (For a basic definition of prayer, see Chapter 4.)

THE CEREMONIAL ACTS: CHANTING, PRAYING, SMUDGING, AND DRINKING HERBAL TEAS

The request for the elders to gather for prayer (which may be said or chanted), smudging, and sipping herbal teas is based on TMH's nature-based "pharmacopeia." Smudging is the burning of medicinal plants, including the four sacred plants (cedar, sage, sweetgrass, and tobacco), with the belief that the smoke produced will result in a cleansing of negative energies. The use of herbal teas is a long-standing custom among tribal groups, and it is the most challenging from the standpoint of medical acceptance. Psychedelic substances may not be the most appropriate for Ted while in a hospital setting; however, a vast number of medicinal herbal teas could substitute for the psychedelic varietals. A friendly dialogue with the patient, family, and fellow elder should result in a constructive collaboration regarding the use of more innocuous teas.

THE SPECIAL OBJECTS CONSIDERED "RITUALISTIC" OR "SACRED": THE DREAMCATCHER

The request for a dreamcatcher reflects the Native American belief that stems from some early oral traditions in which a medicine man/woman prescribed the use of this ornamented net to filter out bad dreams and energies and provide protection to the individual from ill-fated interactions with their environment. In reality, dreamcatchers are widely available commercially in Western society even though many folks who have them do not necessarily understand their origin. In this case, the hanging of the dreamcatcher is straightforward. It will help lessen the level of stress and fears of the patient, and it carries no untoward effects because it is a contactless ornamental measure.

CASE RESOLUTION

Regarding the risk-to-benefit assessment, the approach to a sound decision that harmonizes both allopathic and traditional medical approaches is in order. This patient's requests are typical for a healing ceremony and, except for the use of a psychedelic substance, should not raise eyebrows, considering that an analogous request from a Christian, Jewish, or other religious patient for communion, readings of the Torah, and so on would almost certainly be allowed.

A TMH ceremony typically includes one or more elders, family members, and community members who pray or chant together while sipping herbal tea. In this case, only the type of tea calls for careful dialogue and discernment between the allopathic professionals and the tribal elders. It is reasonable to assume that any psychedelic substance, not properly identified and sanctioned by the hospital's pharmacy or duly prescribed to the patient, should not be allowed. The same is true for alcoholic beverages and other restricted recreational substances.

An open dialog about the risks and the need for not allowing this type of substance is in order. A natural herbal tea, chosen in mutual accord with the health care team, could be appropriate, with the hope and reassurance that once the elder is stabilized and released from the hospital or to hospice, he will be in a state of health that allows for his reintegration to his community and his practices. Finally, the request for a larger room or space is not unheard of, considering the communal nature of tribal social interactions. However, this request may not be easy to accommodate. Notwithstanding, it should be feasible to at least accommodate a few close family and community members, which will make the healing ceremony valid in the eyes of Ted.

KEY POINTS TO REMEMBER

- At the heart of Native American spirituality and healing practices is a deep sense of communing with the environment, nature, and the greater community. It is this interconnection that brings a much-needed sense of being cared for and valued as an important participant in the life of the tribal community at large.
- For Native Americans, wellness and healing are directly interwoven with family, tribal members, nature at large, and the spirit world. Therefore, it is vital for a patient such as Ted to partake of healing interventions that are communal and rooted in their own traditions.

TMH is a transgenerational, multidisciplinary therapeutic processes rooted in the traditions of the first Americans and deeply ingrained in the psychological make-up of tribal members. Therefore, tribal interactions are vital to the emotional and spiritual solace of native American palliative care patients.
Health care providers with Western allopathic medicine training may not fully understand the basis for some of the TMH interventions, but a sympathetic and open attitude to accommodate tribal practices will greatly enhance the quality of life of patients with advanced, chronic, or terminal illness.

References

1. Eisenberger NI. The pain of social disconnection: Examining the shared neural underpinnings of physical and social pain. *Nat Rev Neurosci.* 2012;13(6):421–434. https://doi.org/10.1038/nrn3231
2. Illueca M, Bradshaw YS, Carr DB. Spiritual pain: A symptom in search of a clinical definition. *J Relig Health.* 2023;62:1920–1932. https://doi.org/10.1007/s10 943-022-01645-y

Further Reading

Borchers AT, Keen CL, Stern JS, Gershwin ME. Inflammation and Native American medicine: The role of botanicals. *Am J Clin Nutr.* 2000;72(2):339–347. https://doi. org/10.1093/ajcn/72.2.339
Cohen KS. *Honoring the Medicine: The Essential Guide to Native American Healing.* Random House; 2018.
Koithan M, Farrell C. Indigenous Native American healing traditions. *J Nurse Pract.* 2010;6(6):477–478. https://doi.org/10.1016/j.nurpra.2010.03.016
National Institutes of Health. NIH strategic plan for tribal health research 2019–2023. 2024.https://dpcpsi.nih.gov/sites/default/files/2019_THRO_StrategicPlan_508.pdf
National Institutes of Health. NIH Traditional Medicine Summit report 2019. 2019. https://dpcpsi.nih.gov/sites/default/files/NIH-THRO-2019-Traditional-Medicine-Summit-Report.pdf

9 Dying Alone

Sharon Kim

Mr. C takes pride in being a healthy person. He exercises daily, has a healthy diet, and works extremely hard as the sole income provider for his wife and three children. He has done everything right. As the COVID-19 pandemic disrupted the entire world, he took every recommended precaution to protect himself and his family. Despite these measures, he started exhibiting symptoms. No one could have predicted that this healthy 35-year-old man would land in the intensive care unit (ICU) 3 weeks later requiring a ventilator, subsequently developing multi-organ failure. Mrs. C is dismayed. Due to stringent visitor restrictions, it has been more than a month since she has been able to touch or see Mr. C. She tries to make sense of his critical condition by barely piecing together the overwhelming information she has received through her daily phone updates from various health care staff. And now, the doctors are telling her that he is dying. Overwhelmed by shock and disbelief, she begs the ICU staff for her and their three young children to be able to see him and say their goodbyes. Current hospital policy does not allow for visitors of patients in the ICU confirmed or suspected to be COVID-19 positive.

What do you do now?

DISCUSSION

The World Health Organization declared COVID-19 as a pandemic on March 11, 2020. As the virus rapidly spread at an alarming rate with the potential to cause lethal complications, the entire world seemed to shut down in an attempt to slow the spread. Schools and businesses were closed, flights were canceled, and people were asked to isolate at home as fear and uncertainty ensued. Hospitals were inundated with patients in respiratory distress, leading to a shortage of ICU beds, health care staff, personal protective equipment (PPE), and ventilators. With the unpredictability of the virus and limited resources, hospital systems were forced to place strict isolation precautions and visitor restrictions of varying degrees to prevent further transmission and protect the patients and staff. As a result, patients were disconnected from their families and support systems.

Isolation can have both physical and psychological repercussions. Quarantine for even short durations (<10 days) has been shown to have a psychological toll and is associated with higher risk of acute stress disorder, depression, anxiety, post-traumatic stress disorder, and other mental health issues.[1] Furthermore, loneliness and social isolation can lead to increased mortality risk from all causes.[2] Isolation at the end of life can be especially distressing.

The concept of dying alone is a common unsettling fear shared by most, which became an unfortunate reality for far too many patients during the pandemic. As more of society is recognizing the importance of "dying well," more people are able to envision a peaceful death surrounded by the ones they love. We often hear accounts of actively dying patients waiting for specific loved ones to be bedside before taking their last breath. A study assessing the end-of-life wishes of advanced cancer patients found that the presence of family was of the highest importance second to spirituality.[3] Family members of critically ill patients also prioritize being physically close to their loved ones when in the ICU.[4] Being unable to honor these wishes causes suffering not only to the patient but also to the patient's family and health care staff.

In normal circumstances, families are encouraged to spend as much time as possible with their loved ones who are dying. The majority of families wish to be present with their loved ones at the moment of death and find it important to be able to say their "goodbyes."[5] Thus, not being able to have meaningful communication between the patient and family members prior to the patient's death can be associated with higher rates of depression and complicated grief.[5] This can leave the bereaved family members feeling powerless and abandoned.[6]

In a time of fear and uncertainty with the COVID-19 pandemic, quarantine and isolation were deemed necessary despite possible negative consequences. Identifying the sequelae of the pandemic isolation protocols is essential in establishing future evidence-based isolation policies. This also helps determine better modalities to support the bereaved family members both before and after a patient dies. It has been proposed that more effective communication between the family and the health care staff, performance of essential rituals important to the patient and family at the end of life, and bereavement support after a patient's death can potentially improve a family member's experience and ultimately prevent longer term impacts on the bereaved family.[6]

CASE RESOLUTION

The care team works with the ICU nursing supervisor to advocate for Mrs. C and her children to be allowed to visit the patient. After discussion with hospital administration, Mrs. C is given permission to spend time with Mr. C because it is determined that he is imminently dying. She arrives at the ICU with her children. The ICU physician sits down with her in a quiet room to review the patient's current condition and poor prognosis. She is offered support from social work and spiritual care. She quietly sobs as she processes the overwhelming information presented before her. After several minutes, she walks out of the room and is given instructions on proper PPE use before she is reunited with her husband for the first time in more than a month. Her children are not permitted in their father's room, but they observe from behind the glass doors. They appear confused by their almost unrecognizable father, who is connected to multiple tubes, lines, and machines. They watch Mrs. C as she says her final goodbye while tightly holding his hand.

- Social isolation and feelings of loneliness have both physical and psychological consequences.
- Patients value the presence of their loved ones at end of life.
- Isolation at end of life can intensify suffering.
- Further investigation is required to develop standardized isolation policies while mitigating the potential negative impact of isolation.
- Continued bereavement support for the family, including children, after a patient dies can be beneficial to the grieving process.

References

1. Brooks SK, Webster RK, Smith LE, et al. The psychological impact of quarantine and how to reduce it: Rapid review of the evidence. *Lancet.* 2020;395(10227):912–920. doi:10.1016/s0140-6736(20)30460-8

2. Pantell M, Rehkopf D, Jutte D, Syme SL, Balmes J, Adler N. Social isolation: A predictor of mortality comparable to traditional clinical risk factors. *Am J Public Health.* 2013;103(11):2056–2062. doi:10.2105/AJPH.2013.301261

3. Delgado-Guay MO, Rodriguez-Nunez A, De la Cruz V., et al. Advanced cancer patients' reported wishes at the end of life: A randomized controlled trial. *Support Care Cancer.* 2016;24:4273–4281. https://doi.org/10.1007/s00 520-016-3260-9

4. Jacob M, Horton C, Rance-Ashley S, et al. Needs of patients' family members in an intensive care unit with continuous visitation. *Am J Crit Care.* 2016;25:118–25. doi:10.4037/ajcc2016258

5. Otani H, Yoshida S, Morita T, et al. Meaningful communication before death, but not present at the time of death itself, is associated with better outcomes on measures of depression and complicated grief among bereaved family members of cancer patients. *J Pain Symptom Manage.* 2017;54(3):273–279. doi:10.1016/ j.jpainsymman.2017.07.010

6. Kentish-Barnes N, Cohen-Solal Z, Morin L, Souppart V, Pochard F, Azoulay E. Lived experiences of family members of patients with severe COVID-19 who died in intensive care units in France. *JAMA Network Open.* 2021;4(6):e2113355. doi:10.1001/jamanetworkopen.2021.13355

Further Reading

Ann-Yi S, Azhar A, Bruera E. Dying alone during a pandemic. *J Palliat Med.* 2021;24(12):1905–1908. doi:10.1089/jpm.2020.0718

Buecker S, Horstmann K. Loneliness and social isolation during the COVID-19 pandemic: A systematic review enriched with empirical evidence from a large-scale diary study. *Eur Psychologist.* 2021;26(6):272–284. doi:10.1027/1016-9040/a000453

O'Sullivan R, Burns A, Leavey G, et al. Impact of the COVID-19 pandemic on loneliness and social isolation: A multi-country study. *Int J Environ Res Public Health.* 2021;18(19):9982. https://doi.org/10.3390/ijerph18199982

Schluter PJ, Généreux M, Landaverde E, et al. An eight country cross-sectional study of the psychosocial effects of COVID-19 induced quarantine and/or isolation during the pandemic. *Sci Rep.* 2022;12:13175. https://doi.org/10.1038/s41598-022-16254-8

Wissmath B, Mast FW, Kraus F, Weibel D. Understanding the psychological impact of the COVID-19 pandemic and containment measures: An empirical model of stress. *PLoS One.* 2021;16(7):e0254883. https://doi.org/10.1371/journal.pone.0254883

PART II

Dilemmas Related to Families

10 Navigating Familial Conflict Regarding Information Sharing

Nafiisah B. M. H. Rajabalee and
S. Ian Borison

Mrs. Z is a 59-year-old woman with multiple comorbidities who established care with your clinic last week. She moved to the United States a few months ago, after her husband passed away in her home country of Uzbekistan. Her daughter, Aida, is a radiologist in the same hospital system.

On the initial visit, Mrs. Z was having vague abdominal pain. Examination findings were concerning for ascites. Blood work and imaging were ordered. The findings on the computed tomography scan of the abdomen/pelvis were consistent with metastatic ovarian cancer. Her blood work showed elevated tumor markers, supporting this diagnosis. She was also noted to have significant renal impairment.

Mrs. Z does not speak English and had previously requested that Dr. Aida be called for all results and discussions. You call Dr. Aida and share the difficult news. She is understandably distraught and asks the team not to disclose anything to her mother at her appointment tomorrow.

What do you do now?

DISCUSSION

Serious news is inherently emotionally charged. It is crucial to support patients and families in these vulnerable moments, which are opportunities for human connection. When requests for nondisclosure happen, providers may experience distress and emotional burden. Taking a step back to become actively self-aware and situationally aware helps providers approach these requests with a patient- and family-centered mindset.

Self-awareness refers to the objective process of consciously noting our thoughts and emotions without judgment. It is helpful to pause in emotionally charged situations, breathe, and ask, "What am I feeling right now?" The process of noticing and naming a feeling can help us acknowledge it without feeling paralyzed by it. Furthermore, introspection can help us approach the request with an open mind and negotiate what the next best step will be. It can help let go of "must be's" or "should be's." For instance, the clinician may think,

> If it were me, I would rather know I only have limited time, so I can make the most of it. It is normal to be sad and aggrieved. I can help them with emotional support and our team can be there for them. If only I could let them know this.

Noticing these thoughts and the associated feelings can in turn prime the clinician to be compassionate and empathetic, knowing that the family members also have their own perspectives. In addition, we can recognize elements of countertransference (identifying with the patient or family member). This step helps elicit their thought process while making them feel heard and validated. Thereafter, we can more aptly express the common caring factor as the negotiation proceeds.

Situational awareness is becoming cognizant of what we bring into a room, with appreciation of all other members and factors involved while leaving room for blind spots. Using observation, empathy, and genuine curiosity to understand their perspectives is essential to building a therapeutic alliance. Delivering information in a way the patient prefers is crucial. Some patients may never be ready to hear any information, and that is their right. We can recognize that the headline of a serious news disclosure can stay with us for a lifetime. If we have been recipients of serious news, we can appreciate how a genuinely caring physician is able to make us feel supported.

There are many reasons why loved ones may ask a clinician to withhold information from a patient. Frequently, these requests come from a place of care and desire to protect loved ones from emotional turmoil. Current medical education in the United States focuses on the patient's right to self-determination, autonomy, and truth-telling. Although the request for nondisclosure sometimes seems opposed to the bioethical principles that guide many clinicians' practice, this is not always the case.

Some requests for nondisclosure emanate from cultural norms. Culture can strongly influence a patient's information and medical decision-making preferences. In some cultures, discussing life-limiting illnesses or death is considered harmful to the patient. Some cultures place the responsibility of decision-making on family members. Within the same culture, however, variation among each individual's acceptance of cultural norms exists. Therefore, it is important to keep an open mind, explore preferences, and avoid generalizing.

We propose a five-step patient- and family-centered approach to this communication shown in Figure 10.1. First, we suggest clarifying the reasoning behind the request with nonconfrontational language—for example, "I can see how much you care for your mother. May I ask why you suggest we hold off telling her?" This understanding equips us to address the concerns.

Once the reasons driving this request are clarified, we proceed to validation. If familial beliefs or cultural norms govern the nondisclosure of medical information, it is important to validate these requests. If the family member believes the disclosure could be detrimental to the patient's health, it is appropriate to normalize these concerns.

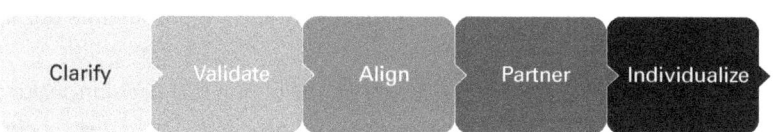

FIGURE 10.1 A five-step approach to navigating requests for non-disclosure.

Now that the family member's concerns have been elicited and validated, we can align and partner with the family member—for instance, by stating,

We are here to support your mother and your family through this. We want to honor her wishes. I hear that your mother expects you to receive information and make medical decisions on her behalf. Let us discuss with her the possibility of you serving as her surrogate for her medical care."

When there is a language barrier, it is very important to use qualified interpretation services, especially when discussing information preferences and potential surrogacy. Although some patients may decline interpretation services and prefer family members to interpret, situations such as these necessitate an objective third party. It is often helpful to highlight that the use of an interpreter helps relieve an additional burden so that they can focus on being a family member. Interpretation also amplifies the patient's voice, which is important when deciding on a surrogate.

The final step is to individualize the plan in accordance with the patient's wishes. If the patient requests disclosure of all health-related information and to maintain their right to decision-making, this should be honored. Similarly, if the patient elects to have their information delivered to a trusted surrogate and rely on a loved one for medical decision-making, this should likewise be honored. This is in alignment with autonomy, a fundamental principle in bioethics.

In the pragmatic sense, every clinical scenario involves unique patient circumstances. Cultural humility acknowledges that patients and families are experts in their own values.[1-3] It highlights the fact that clinicians' thought processes are not always right and respectfully supports the patient/family amid disagreements.[1-3]

Autonomy is a fundamental principle of bioethics. A patient can defer that right to a trusted person of their choice to act on their behalf. Some cultures consider the whole family as a unit who can act on behalf of the sick person without burdening the patient with such responsibilities during their vulnerable moments.

The principle of truth-telling hinges on the notion that decision-making necessitates full understanding of the clinical situation. The patient, being autonomous, can opt for not knowing and choose a surrogate to be the recipient of information. The principle of truth-telling is still honored if the medical information is shared with the chosen surrogate instead.

All patient/family requests are opportunities for human interaction and if viewed as such can alleviate some of the associated hesitation, discomfort, and anguish. Serious illnesses are moments of vulnerability. Navigating requests for nondisclosures will remain challenging. However, we can approach them with an open mind, listen intently, and utilize some of the above communication framework to guide these situations.

CASE RESOLUTION

We meet Mrs. Z and Dr. Aida in clinic the next day. Mrs. Z greets you warmly and looks weaker than last week. She tells you, with the help of a medical interpreter, that she feels her abdominal pain is "not as bad" these days. Dr. Aida has a stoic look on her face. She asks to speak to the team outside the room. The team asks Mrs. Z if it is okay to speak with Dr. Aida separately outside of the room, and she agrees.

The physician offers a seat to Dr. Aida and pauses and allows her to speak. The physician listens empathetically: Dr. Aida tells the team that her mother has always been a strong woman and that she has a strong faith. She does not want her already bereaved mother to receive "another piece of hard news as of yet." Dr. Aida states she already knows that her mother's metastatic cancer is not amenable to palliative debulking surgery. She worries any chemotherapy will not add any mortality benefit. She states that her mother is her only parent left.

The physician notices that she can relate to Aida and relives some moments of a similar situation when her own aunt was diagnosed with metastatic colon cancer. She cannot recall the headline the surgeon had said, but she remembers feeling frozen. She can notice her own sadness and the one she feels with the difficult situation both Mrs. Z and her daughter are in. She exercises social awareness and cultural humility as she leans in and asks Dr. Aida about her reasoning.

The tone of the physician's voice indicates care, as does the associated body language. The physician asks curious questions about their values to define and discover the reasons of information withholding. Dr. Aida shares that as Mrs. Z's only daughter and as a physician, her mother trusts and expects her to handle all aspects of her health care. She conveys that she worries about sharing the news of this diagnosis, especially if there are no disease-directed treatment options; it would only cause her mother unnecessary psychological distress. Following the discussion, Dr. Aida agrees to be present with the physician to ask her mother about her preferences for information sharing and decision-making. Mrs. Z indicates, with the help of an interpreter, that she would like to let Dr. Aida receive all prognostic information and to act as a surrogate for medical decisions.

The physician organizes a multidisciplinary team meeting the next day with the oncologist, the social worker, and Dr. Aida. Mrs. Z decides to let her daughter attend the meeting on her behalf. The team discusses that the risks of chemotherapy likely outweigh the benefits with her current renal impairment and functional status. The care team decides to focus Mrs. Z's care on her comfort.

During the next 2 months, Mrs. Z stays at home with her daughter and grandchildren. Her pain is well managed by hospice services. Mrs. Z dies at home. The physician meets Dr. Aida later, and she expresses gratefulness.

KEY POINTS TO REMEMBER

- Requests for nondisclosure can cause distress for clinicians. Focusing on self-awareness and situational awareness allows for an open-minded response.
- Every discussion can begin with agreeing that every person in the care unit—the patient, family members, and clinicians—has the best interest of the patient in mind.
- Before directly addressing a request for nondisclosure, clarify the reasons driving the request.
- We propose using a five-step approach to these requests by focusing on clarifying, validating, aligning, partnering, and individualizing.
- When facing a language barrier, it is crucial to utilize appropriate interpretation services, particularly when discussing patients'

preferences regarding information sharing and medical decision-making.

- We can navigate negotiations using a nonviolent communication framework and thereafter scaffolding individual elements in.
- Interdisciplinary team members can bring additional skill sets to support discussions as they unfold.

References

1. MacKenzie L, Hatala A. Addressing culture within healthcare settings: The limits of cultural competence and the power of humility. *Can Med Educ J.* 2019;10(1):e124–e127. https://pubmed.ncbi.nlm.nih.gov/30949267

2. Masters C, Robinson D, Faulkner S, et al. Addressing biases in patient care with the 5Rs of cultural humility, a clinician coaching tool. *J Gen Intern Med.* 2019;34(4):627–630. https://doi.org/10.1007/s11606-018-4814-y

3. McGee-Avila J. Practicing cultural humility to transform health care. Robert Wood Johnson Foundation. 2018. https://www.rwjf.org/en/blog/2018/06/practicing-cultu ral-humility-to-transform-healthcare.html

Further Reading

Chen-Stokes S, Pan C. Health and health care of Chinese American older adults. eCampus Geriatrics. 2010. http://geriatrics.stanford.edu/wp-content/uploads/ downloads/ethnomed/chinese/downloads/chinese_american.pdf

Choudry M, Latif AA, Warburton KG. An overview of the spiritual importances of end-of-life care among the five major faiths of the United Kingdom. *Clin Med.* 2018;18(1):23–31. https://doi.org/10.7861/clinmedicine.18-1-23

de Pentheny O'Kelly C, Urch C, Brown EA. The impact of culture and religion on truth telling at the end of life. *Nephrol Dial Transplant.* 2011;26(12):3838–3842. https:// doi.org/10.1093/ndt/gfr630

Lee J. *Talking Across the Divide.* Penguin; 2018.

Leng J, Lui F, Chen A, et al. Adapting meaning-centered psychotherapy in advanced cancer for the Chinese immigrant population. *J Immigr Minor Health.* 2018;20(3):680–686. https://doi.org/10.1007/s10903-017-0591-7

Liu Y, Yang J, Huo D, et al. Disclosure of cancer diagnosis in China: The incidence, patients' situation, and different preferences between patients and their family members and related influence factors. *Cancer Manag Res.* 2018;10:2173–2181. https://doi.org/10.2147/CMAR.S166437

Pergert P, Lützén K. Balancing truth-telling in the preservation of hope: A relational ethics approach. *Nurs Ethics*. 2012;19(1):21–29. https://doi.org/10.1177/096973301 1418551

Rosenburg MB. *Nonviolent Communication: A Language of Life*. 2nd ed. Puddledancer Press; 2005.

Seo B. *Good Arguments*. Penguin; 2023.

Zolkefli Y. The ethics of truth-telling in health-care settings. *Malays J Med Sci*. 2018;25(3):135–139. https://doi.org/10.21315/mjms2018.25.3.14

11 Dis/Continuing Transfusions in a 2-Year-Old Dying of Leukemia

Elizabeth Pasternak and Pamela Ressler

Your 2-year-old patient with leukemia is dying in the pediatric intensive care unit (PICU). Her parents want to continue transfusions.

What do you do now?

DISCUSSION

Parents play a key role in decision-making for treatment for their child and need to be part of shared goal setting throughout the illness. In the case presented here, is there a misalignment with the clinical team with goals of care? Have the parents been asked what they hope the transfusions will bring to their daughter's treatment/care?

During the past few decades, the cure rate for pediatric malignancies has improved considerably. However, nearly 20% of pediatric patients with cancer still die from their disease. Many will die in the acute care setting rather than at home with hospice care. The parents of children with cancer report that end-of-life decisions are the most difficult treatment-related decisions that they face during the children's cancer experience. ICUs at children's hospitals are increasingly occupied by chronically critically ill children. Decisions surrounding initiation, continuation, escalation, or de-escalation of life-prolonging interventions frequently occur in these units. In reality, the goals and priorities of the health care system are not always in alignment with those of whom the system serves. Distress can be palpable when staff perceive that decisions in the best interest of these children and their families are not always being made. The literature acknowledges that optimizing the quality of medical care given at the end of life is an important health care objective. Priority should be placed on relieving the child's end-of-life distress, with consideration of the long-lasting implications for the bereaved parents, who will be negatively affected by their child's experience of unmanageable symptoms years after the child's death.

As patient- and family-centered care becomes an increasingly integral component of modern medicine, it is important for health care to partner with parents and guardians, recognizing that they often possess valuable knowledge and life experience regarding their child. The ability of providers to embrace a patient-centered culture empowers parents to have voice in the management and delivery of their child's care. The literature suggests that parental involvement in decision-making of their hospitalized child leads to an improvement in quality of care and patient safety.

Regarding the case presented in this chapter, it is vital for you to explore with the parents the significance and meaning behind why they wish for their child to continue to receive transfusions. During the course of their daughter's illness, transfusions may have been perceived as a lifeline by her parents. At the time of diagnosis, the parents were likely counseled in great detail about how leukemia is different from many cancers in that there is no tumor; rather, the cancerous cells are found throughout the body, in the blood or in bone marrow. They have witnessed firsthand how leukemia interferes with the normal production of red cells, white cells, and platelets. It would have been common for their daughter to have developed anemia (low levels of red cells) and thrombocytopenia (low levels of platelets), which on several occasions may have warranted transfusions. It is important for the health care team(s) and parents to have a discussion about the implication of continued blood transfusions at this current stage of illness: What do the parents hope that the blood transfusions will provide? Do the parents fear that their daughter will bleed to death? Do they worry that she will suffer? Does stopping transfusions mean that they are giving up? Are they hoping for more time or waiting for a miracle? Are they worried that their daughter will experience symptoms—after all, they have witnessed her become anemic in the past, which always resulted in transfusions. Did they have a bad experience with a loved one dying in the past? What have they heard from others (friends, family, and clinicians) or seen on television?

CASE RESOLUTION

To stratify communication between the interdisciplinary team and family, you arrange a team meeting with the child's parents and key members of the health care team to discuss blood transfusions for the child.

Talking about goals of care is the pivotal communication task when you are caring for a child with a serious illness. Your willingness to meet with the family is hugely important, especially when decisions need to be considered, and you want to support constructive coping. During the team meeting, it is important to first elicit what the parents understand of their daughter's medical situation. You need to establish a degree of understanding before moving the conversation forward. A number of strategies and frameworks are helpful when having these conversations. The mnemonic REMAP can be a framework to help guide you in goals of care conversations.

REMAP stands for *re*frame, *e*xpect emotion, *m*ap out patient/family values, *a*lign with goals, and *p*ropose a plan:

Reframe: Assess the parent's understanding of their daughter's expected illness trajectory and, if necessary, provide new information. This places the details of their daughter's illness into a bigger picture known as the "headline" and lets the parents know that aspects of their daughter's illness have changed. This helps justify the need to re-evaluate the goals of care for their daughter. Using a preamble such as "We are worried that . . ." or "I think that . . ." will also allow you to provide the medical impression without claiming absolute knowledge of the future. Of note, it is not necessary for the parents to accept the medical view of their daughter's prognosis to continue the conversation. In fact, many parents doubt clinicians' prognostic estimates. Should there be disagreement, explore the parent's view of the situation. Again, intersect open-ended questions, such as "What you are thinking?" Experts suggest that empathizing with the parents can be more helpful than repeating the prognostic information. In an effort to allow parents to hold hope for the best outcome for their daughter while still engaging in a contingency plan should things worsen, you might say,

> We understand that you feel it is important to maintain a sense of optimism. We will do everything that we can to optimize your daughter's care. We are wondering if you could also think about the possibility that things might not work out as we hope.

Expect emotion: Next, pause and embrace the emotional response. It would not be surprising if the parents displayed a reaction to thinking about their daughter's disease progression and/or the idea that she could die during this hospitalization. At this point, you could consider asking the parents for permission to move forward with the conversation. For example, "Would it be alright for us to talk more about what this means for your daughter's future?"

Map out patient/family values: To help map parental goals, you need to continue to ask open-ended questions to help elicit their values that should ultimately guide their daughter's treatment. You should intentionally explore the parent's values before discussing any therapeutic choices. One approach might include stating, "In order to figure out the best plan for your daughter, let's spend some time talking about what is most important to you and your family during this time." Perhaps the parents would like to bring a sibling to visit or a family pet. Do they want to engage in legacy making?

Align with goals: To align with the parents' expressed values, explicitly reflect them back. This allows for more of a reflection and summary of the conversation. Should parents give you a sign that they are ready to transition into the planning phase or grant you permission, you can then use those values to propose a medical plan that ideally matches their values. Should the parents not ask for a plan, you might need to invest more time exploring and clarifying or could ask a follow-up question such as "Would it be okay if our team shares with you our recommendation?" The plan should start with what will be done to achieve the parent's goals. During the discussion, it is also applicable to share with the parents what you think will not achieve their expressed goals.

Propose a plan: Parents are often fierce advocates for their children and believe that it is their responsibility to decide what is best for their child—deferring a need to receive a medical recommendation. In such instances, you can continue to ask open-ended questions to explore how you can best assist the parents with decision-making: Tell me what you are thinking about the next steps? What are you hoping for? What are you worried about? How can I/my team be most helpful to you and your family during this time? This process requires you to seek understanding, remain flexible, and adapt your recommendations based on what you hear from the parents and/or other specialists involved. Ongoing revisions may be necessary. Ultimately, this will lead to family-centered decision-making that promotes better end-of-life care.

In our case, the health care team uses the REMAP framework in several conversations with the patient's parents and comes to understand the parents' belief that blood transfusions have helped their daughter with symptom management in the past. They value keeping their daughter as symptom-free as possible for as long as possible. A discussion follows, with team members and the parents deciding that they are in need of expanded palliative care resources at this point in the daughter's disease. A plan is put in place to continue to use transfusions on a limited basis, in consultation with the palliative care team, for the purpose of symptom management. Prioritizing symptom management with a variety of interventions for the child and family becomes the primary goal of care.

KEY POINTS TO REMEMBER

- Patient- and family-centered care is an integral component of modern medicine.
- Emphasize respect for values in individual care decisions as well as the role of patients and families as advisors and partners in improving care practice throughout all stages of illness.
- Continue to assess goals of care if and when clinical status changes, there is worry that interventions are no longer effective, or initiating new interventions will be nonbeneficial.
- Understanding of and expectations for the course of illness or particular interventions may differ between parents and clinicians. Allow opportunities to discuss, clarify, and provide resources and recommendations as necessary.
- Use clinical tools such as REMAP to aid in values-guided decision-making about treatment decisions.

Further Reading

1. Aarthun A, Øymar KA, Akerjordet K. Parental involvement in decision-making about their child's health care at the hospital. *Nurs Open*. 2018;6(1):50–58. doi:10.1002/nop2.180
2. Latha SM, Scott JX, Kumar S, Kumar SM, Subramanian L, Rajendran A. Parent's perspectives on the end-of-life care of their child with cancer: Indian perspective. *Indian J Palliat Care*. 2016;22(3):317–325. doi:10.4103/0973-1075.185047
3. Childers JW, Back AL, Tulsky JA, Arnold RM. REMAP: A framework for goals of care conversations. *J Oncol Pract*. 2017;13(10):e844–e850.
4. ACT. Making critical care choices. March 2017. https://api.courageousparentsnetwork.org/app/uploads/2016/02/ACT_MakingCriticalCareChoices.pdf

5. Courageous Parents Network. Shared decision-making. 2022. https://api.coura geousparentsnetwork.org/app/uploads/2022/05/Shared-Decision-Making-5.22.pdf
6. Kim JY, Park BK. The most important aspects for a good death: Perspectives from parents of children with cancer. *INQUIRY*. 2021;58. doi:10.1177/ 00469580211028580
7. Virtual Hospice. Cancer. 2024. https://www.virtualhospice.ca/en_US/Main+Site+ Navigation/Home/Support/Support/Asked+and+Answered/What+to+Expect+ with+Various+Illnesses/Cancer/What+can+be+expected+as+leukemia+progress es_.aspx
8. VitalTalk. VitalTalk courses. 2024. https://www.chooseyourpath.vitaltalk.org

Recommended Resources

Courageous Parents Network (https://courageousparentsnetwork.org) is a non-profit organization and educational platform that orients, empowers, and accompanies families and providers caring for children with serious illness.

VitalTalk (https://www.chooseyourpath.vitaltalk.org) provides communication training for those working with patients with serious illness.

12 Managing Family Conflict

Betty R. Ferrell

Aunt Martha's family complains that she "makes everything into a big deal" just so she can be consoled by everyone that everything will be OK after she passes. But we (health care professionals) do not think they will be OK. The family members bicker among themselves about inheritances and argue who is empowered to make medical decisions for her. In addition, the family has been in chronic turmoil for years, and half of them do not talk to the other half.

Aunt Martha's breast cancer has recurred, and she is now experiencing renal failure and heart failure after completing chemotherapy. She has begun to experience confusion and rapid physical decline. Her family and support systems include a close friend Beatrice; her ex-spouse, Carl; a nephew George, who has a history of severe depression; and a niece Alice, who has been estranged for many years. None seem to agree on what is best for Aunt Martha.

What do you do now?

DISCUSSION

A core value of the field of palliative care is family-centered care. Clinicians in palliative care settings value psychosocial support and family involvement in care, and they view family caregivers as "secondary patients" who need support throughout an illness and through bereavement.

These essential values, however, are often tested in the real world of patient and family care, in which relationships are often fractured, motives are questionable, and decades of conflict seem to come to a tumultuous eruption as illness progresses and death is near. In these times of family conflict, palliative care clinicians should consider strategies that will best serve the patient, often at the center of the family conflict, and preserve the integrity of the team. They should avoid becoming engulfed by often decades of family history that can easily overshadow the patient nearing death.

Several authors have described strategies for managing family conflict and maintaining the focus on the needs of the patient and the goals of care. All agree that use of an interdisciplinary team is essential.[1–9] Studies have documented the impact of family conflict on patient safety; loss of trust in the clinicians; communication conflicts; and ill effects on the patient, such as withdrawal or depression. Sources also document that cultural conflicts are often at the center of these situations and the need for culturally respectful care.

Other factors common in these difficult family situations include lack of understanding the prognosis and goals of care. Early use of family conferencing and enlisting the support of psychosocial services are critical. Caregivers of older adults, those with high caregiver burden or financial challenges, and families with previous mental health concerns are high risk for conflict as the patient nears the end of life.[1,7,8] Ashana and colleagues[2] describe application of principles of "trauma-informed care," including attention to patient safety, trustworthiness and transparency, collaboration and peer support, and empowerment and other means to provide family support. They describe training for clinicians in skills of negotiation and dispute resolution to manage conflicts. Zaider and colleagues[9] provide direction for teaching clinicians communication skills to apply to these situations.

CASE RESOLUTION

Aunt Martha's family conflicts become even more intense as her disease progresses. Upon learning that Aunt Martha has left her estate to her neighbor, her nephew, niece, and ex-spouse insist that she start dialysis against her objections to provide time so they can seek legal assistance and persuade Martha to change her will.

Martha's clinical team engages an ethics consultation and social work consult to address the family conflicts so that they can remain focused on Martha's care, including her escalating physical symptoms and the need to arrange inpatient hospice placement to provide a peaceful environment for her death.

Through the assistance of the team, ethicist, and social worker, Martha's friend Beatrice is named her health care proxy, and she is able to honor Martha's goals of care as Martha dies in hospice.

KEY POINTS TO REMEMBER

- Palliative care is family-focused care, yet clinicians also may need to prioritize the best interests of the patient.
- Family conflicts and dysfunction likely have a long history preceding the current illness of the patient and are unlikely to resolve in the face of illness progression and death. The dysfunction may get worse.
- Complex family dynamics and conflicts are best addressed by an interdisciplinary team and may also require consultation from an ethicist or legal source.
- Amid the escalation of family conflict, emotions, and the resulting chaos, the palliative care team should remain focused on the patient goals of care.

References

1. Alshehry AS. Nurse–patient/relatives conflict and patient safety competence among nurses. *INQUIRY*. 2022;59:469580221093186.
2. Ashana DC, Lewis C, Hart JL. Dealing with "difficult" patients and families: Making a case for trauma-informed care in the intensive care unit. *Ann Am Thorac Soc*. 2020;17(5):541–544.

3. Campbell M, Ramirez-Zohfeld V, Seltzer A, Lindquist LA. Training hospitalists in negotiations to address conflicts with older adults around their social needs. *Geriatrics*. 2020;5(3):50.

4. Laidsaar-Powell R, Butow P, Boyle F, Juraskova I. Managing challenging interactions with family caregivers in the cancer setting: Guidelines for clinicians (TRIO Guidelines–2). *Patient Educ Couns*. 2018;101(6):983–994.

5. Laidsaar-Powell R, Butow P, Boyle F, Juraskova I. Facilitating collaborative and effective family involvement in the cancer setting: Guidelines for clinicians (TRIO Guidelines–1). *Patient Educ Couns*. 2018;101(6):970–982.

6. Laidsaar-Powell R, Keast R, Butow P, et al. Improving breast cancer nurses' management of challenging situations involving family carers: Pilot evaluation of a brief targeted online education module (TRIO–Conflict). *Patient Educ Couns*. 2021;104(12):3023–3031.

7. Laryionava K, Winkler EC. Dealing with family conflicts in decision-making in end-of-life care of advanced cancer patients. *Curr Oncol Rep*. 2021;23(11):124.

8. Mulcahy Symmons S, Ryan K, Aoun SM, et al. Decision-making in palliative care: Patient and family caregiver concordance and discordance—Systematic review and narrative synthesis. *BMJ Support Palliat Care*. 2023;13(4):374–385.

9. Zaider TI, Banerjee SC, Manna R, et al. Responding to challenging interactions with families: A training module for inpatient oncology nurses. *Fam Syst Health*. 2016;34(3):204–212.

13 Dilemmas Related to Families

Anna Barreiro Albán and Beth B. Hogans

A 74-year-old mother has discussed with her husband, children, and granddaughters that in the event of a serious illness and if she is in need of hospice care, she wishes to die at home surrounded by her loved ones. She would like to spend her last days of life focusing on the family unit and the good moments shared with the people she loves. She has expressed preference for quality of life (QoL) rather than extension of life. She has a medical history of hypertension. Once while exercising, she experienced a debilitating headache and was admitted to the emergency room. She was diagnosed with suffering a cryptogenic stroke, which left her depressed and weakened. In addition, she experienced a substantial decline in mobility and a gradual decline in memory and cognition that in time started to interfere with her work performance and activities of daily living. She was referred to the neurologist and diagnosed with Alzheimer's disease and dementia, and she was placed to receive palliative care and hospice care. The mother wants to go home, not to a nursing home. Her husband and children state that they cannot take care of her at home because they have concerns about what to do when she is experiencing agitation, secretions, altered breathing, pain, confusion, and mood and sleep disturbances.

What do you do now?

DISCUSSION

A family caregiver who is caring for a loved one affected by a life-threating illness hopes to provide the best care possible and keep the person safe and comfortable, helping them maintain their autonomy. Caring for a loved one at the end of life is often very emotionally and physically difficult. In many circumstances, it is overwhelming, creating fear, grief, and sometimes disagreement between family members even though affection, affinity, and closeness are still present in the family dynamic. This experience is usually accompanied with conflicting feelings of regret; moral and ethical dilemmas; and anxiety, depression, and the grief of impending loss—expressed and manifested by each family caregiver differently when confronted with having to make critical decisions regarding medical care, in many cases without a complete understanding of the disease diagnosis, prognosis, and supportive care plan, or with insufficient information about palliative care resources and continuity of care. Therefore, it is imperative that health care professionals focus on cultural competence in palliative practice, giving importance to the cultural and spiritual aspects, beliefs, values, and experiences of each patient and family member to whom they provide palliative care services.

To support individualized compassionate patient-centered palliative care, health care practitioners have the ethical obligation to provide the highest quality end-of-life care and anticipate the needs of patients and caregivers, centering their attention on essential components of palliative care medicine, such as illness and prognosis education, symptoms and functional status management, creation of effective communication interventions, and building rapport. Interdisciplinary teams should recognize specific individualized cultural, social, psychological, and spiritual needs of the patients and families because it is crucial to be respectful of cultural norms and beliefs.

Interdisciplinary teams should consider the effects on QoL and well-being by the numerous daily stressors and caregivers' experience when providing home care for a loved one. Research has shown that care demands, which differ with the intensity of care and disease progression, can cause family caregivers different levels of distress. For instance, providing around-the-clock care responsibilities, worrying about the complexity of care activities, the ability to perform and complete care tasks, and feelings of apprehension about dysfunctional change in caregiving activities[1] can increase caregivers' burden. Furthermore, caregivers' burden is related to dependency of the care recipient; illness progression; and severity of the care situation, which increases over the course of the illness, thus affecting caregivers' well-being and health.[1] Duration of family care and the patient's dependency level[2,3] are considered two of the most significant causes of caregivers' burden. Moreover, to improve the quality of support services, it is critical that the care team properly document the planning and implementation of supportive care plans; this is often omitted in nursing care plans and progress notes.[1]

To improve patient- and family-centered palliative care and QoL, it is vital to understand patients' and primary caregivers' emotional experiences. Patients and family caregivers frequently face multiple barriers to the implementation of an integrated model of palliative care that emphasizes individualized needs and collaborative efforts that facilitate improvement of interpersonal communication between the patient, family, and primary and specialty teams. It is important that health care professionals establish honest, compassionate, respectful conversations with the families of patients affected by terminal illnesses. Furthermore, family caregivers need to be considered as part of the care team. Their unique perspectives, intimate knowledge of the patient, and decisions must be integrated in the palliative care plan goals. Family caregivers value compassionate care, respect of patient's individuality and pragmatic expectations,[4] and the patient's autonomy in end-of-life decisions, especially in cases in which they need to protect vulnerable patients who have lost the ability to make decisions due to increased cognitive decline and disease progression.

CASE RESOLUTION

The family is distraught witnessing the progression of the disease and rapid changes observed in cognitive decline. The patient is suffering cardiac complications, aphasia, paralysis, and increased distress. After she is admitted to neuropalliative home care to receive supportive long-term care, the care plan goals are discussed with her husband and daughters. This leads to a conversation between family members in which they express feeling incapable of taking care of her. The family discusses the difficult task of performing continuous caring activities and feeling anxious about completing these tasks properly, in addition to fulfilling the expectations of the health care team and other family members.

The patient's support system is one of her granddaughters, with whom she is very close and has a special relationship. The older granddaughter decides to become the primary caregiver and is happy to fulfill her grandmother's wishes. She is designated as her grandmother's health care proxy. She advocates for her grandmother's wishes, recognizing that she must focus on keeping her grandmother conformable and safe and not on the complexity of the situation and complications of the illness. The family honors the patient's wishes of dying at home with her family. The whole family is reunited, and she dies surrounded by her loved ones. The family effectively communicated and resolved their differences and the dilemma of caring for the patient at home versus a nursing home. All members supported the primary caregiver's decision to honor the patient's wishes. The interdisciplinary team (hospice physician and nurse, social worker, and clergy) met with the family to assess their needs and arrange the care plan, referring them to appropriate resources, acknowledging cultural norms, and aiding in decision-making and symptom management. Moreover, they acted in the best interests of the patient and the family and, most important, practiced compassionate patient-centered palliative care, engaging the patient and caregivers as part of the health care team.

KEY POINTS TO REMEMBER

- Acknowledgment of patients' right to autonomy and individuality
- Empathy for families' complex situations and unique experiences
- Involvement of patients and caregivers as part of interdisciplinary team
- Compassionate understanding of each individual case and family dynamics

- Consideration of patients'/families' personal decisions, religious beliefs and cultural norms, values, perspectives, and experiences
- Recognition of patients' and family caregivers' needs and expectations to help reduce caregiver distress, anxiety, and depression
- Significance of patients'/families' and practitioners' communication in shared decision-making process to improve patient-centered palliative care
- Awareness of detrimental effects of loss and stress, and negative emotional experiences regarding caregivers' well-being

References

1. van Driel AG, Becqué Y, Rietjens JAC, van der Heide A, Witkamp FE. Supportive nursing care for family caregivers: A retrospective nursing file study. *Appl Nurs Res*. 2021;59:151434. doi:10.1016/j.apnr.2021.151434
2. Bijnsdorp FM, Onwuteaka-Philipsen BD, Boot CRL, van der Beek AJ, Pasman HRW. Caregiver's burden at the end of life of their loved one: Insights from a longitudinal qualitative study among working family caregivers. *BMC Palliat Care*. 2022;21(1):142. doi:10.1186/s12904-022-01031-1
3. Lindt N, van Berkel J, Mulder BC. Determinants of overburdening among informal carers: A systematic review. *BMC Geriatr*. 2020;20(1):304. doi:10.1186/s12877-020-01708-3
4. Hill SR, Mason H, Poole M, Vale L, Robinson L. What is important at the end of life for people with dementia? The views of people with dementia and their carers. *Int J Geriatr Psychiatry*. 2016;32(9):1037–1045. doi:10.1002/gps.4564

Further Reading

Bolt SR, Steen JT, Khemai C, Schols JMGA, Zwakhalen SMG, Meijers JMM. The perspectives of people with dementia on their future, end of life and on being cared for by others: A qualitative study. *J Clin Nurs*. 2022;31(13–14):1738–1752. doi:10.1111/jocn.15644

Cain CL, Surbone A, Elk R, Kagawa-Singer M. Culture and palliative care: Preferences, communication, meaning, and mutual decision making. *J Pain Symptom Manage*. 2018;55(5):1408–1419. doi:10.1016/j.jpainsymman.2018.01.007

Givler A, Bhatt H, Maani-Fogelman PA. The importance of cultural competence in pain and palliative care. In *StatPearls*. StatPearls Publishing; 2019. Accessed May 22, 2023. https://www.ncbi.nlm.nih.gov/books/NBK493154

Martín JM, Olano-Lizarraga M, Saracíbar-Razquin M. The experience of family caregivers caring for a terminal patient at home: A research review. *Int J Nurs Stud.* 2016;64:1–12. doi:10.1016/j.ijnurstu.2016.09.010

Michaels J, Chen C, Ann Meeker M. Navigating the caregiving abyss: A metasynthesis of how family caregivers manage end-of-life care for older adults at home. *Palliat Medicine.* 2022;36(1):81–94. https://doi.org/10.1177/0269216321 1042999

Morey T, Scott M, Saunders S, et al. Transitioning from hospital to palliative care at home: Patient and caregiver perceptions of continuity of care. *J Pain Symptom Manage.* 2021;62(2):233–241. doi:10.1016/j.jpainsymman.2020.12.019

Ryan RE, Connolly M, Bradford NK, et al. Interventions for interpersonal communication about end of life care between health practitioners and affected people. *Cochrane Database Syst Rev.* 2022;7(7):CD013116. doi:10.1002/14651858. cd013116.pub2

Thompson GN, Roger K. Understanding the needs of family caregivers of older adults dying with dementia. *Palliat Support Care.* 2013;12(3):223–231. doi:10.1017/ s1478951513000461

14 Complicated Grief

Zhu Wang and Salahadin Abdi

Mr. Smith is a 78-year-old male with metastatic melanoma who was trialed unsuccessfully on numerous standard treatments and clinical trials. Because there are no other treatments available for his cancer, he and his wife of 50 years enrolled him into home hospice. However, he developed worsening of his breathing and became unconscious. His wife called 911 to take him to a local emergency room and revoked his hospice. In the emergency room, they found him to no longer have a pulse, but his wife insisted that cardiopulmonary resuscitation be done. Unfortunately, Mr. Smith was unable to be resuscitated and was pronounced dead in the emergency room. Fifteen months later, Mr. Smith's daughter calls you and expresses that she is concerned about her mother. She tells you that although her father passed away more than 15 months ago, her mother continues to feel sad all the time. Her daughter explains that her mother feels guilty. She also adds that her mother had an episode of depression when she was younger, but it "went away." Now, her mother stays in bed almost all day, eats very little, avoids family events, and cries frequently. The daughter has tried several times to encourage and support her mother, but she is refusing everything.

What do you do now?

DISCUSSION

In this case, Mrs. Smith had lost her husband to cancer and continues to grieve more than a year after his death. Grieving is a normal reaction; however, is it still normal when it is prolonged? When is it considered normal versus abnormal grieving?

Let us consider normal grief first. It was proposed by Dr. Kubler-Ross that there are five stages of normal grief toward the end of life: denial, anger, bargaining, depression, and acceptance[1] Different individuals can experience different stages at different times. Some can skip stages. As suggested in this model, acceptance can be achieved. Progression through these steps is considered to represent normal grieving. After an individual dies, their family members are often in distress, as in the case of Mrs. Smith. However, when an individual is unable to come to terms with their loss, abnormal processes such as complicated grief can arise.

In this case, Mrs. Smith is clearly experiencing grief. It is also apparent that her prolonged sadness has interfered with her daily activities. She is unable to resume her previous life due to the death of her husband more than a year ago. This prolonged grief is considered complicated grief, and it is an abnormal process. By consensus, grief is considered complicated when symptoms persist after 6–12 months of losing their loved one. In the fifth edition of the *Diagnostic and Statistical Manual of Mental Disorders*, it is termed prolonged grief disorder (PGD).[2] PGD is a persistent and pervasive grief response and is accompanied by a number of other symptoms, including intense emotional pain and difficulties with engaging in daily activities.[2] However, it is described as different from major depressive disorder (MDD) because MDD exhibits additional decreased self-worth or suicide ideation or plan.

Many factors can contribute to the development of complicated grief, including insecure attachment, social situations such as disenfranchisement of individuals in the family, past trauma, disease progression, or prior diagnosis of depression.[3,4] In Mrs. Smith's case, there are likely also some components of guilt. She had witnessed an unquestionably traumatic experience with cardiopulmonary resuscitation in the emergency room. She might be feeling guilty for revoking hospice and having her husband go through what he did. This could have been prevented with early discussions of goals of care.

To prevent complicated grief, health care providers should actively facilitate discussions between the patient and their loved ones. This discussion not only helps with the dying process for the patient but also sets the stage for transitioning by their loved ones after the patient's death. Some of the common topics include goals of care at end of life, their love for each other, and spirituality or religious faith. This can also be a time to discuss their feelings of guilt or obtain forgiveness from each other. In Mrs. Smith's case, they would likely have discussed potential transfer back to the hospital and whether Mr. Smith would want resuscitation. Knowing his wishes more clearly, Mrs. Smith would know what to do and would have avoided this traumatic experience and feeling guilty for what her husband had to go through at the end of his life.

It is clear that Mrs. Smith is going through a tough time. She is experiencing complicated grief because her husband died more than 15 months ago. It is always best to prevent any illness, but how do we treat complicated grief? Some recommendations include reducing repeated exposures to belongings of their loved ones, reducing activities such as frequent visits to their graves, and attempts to resume previous activities. If severe, pharmacotherapy could potentially help; however, no studies have proven its benefit. Once the survivor has developed complicated grief, as did Mrs. Smith, it is important to prevent progression into depression, which includes any signs of decreased self-worth or thoughts of suicide. Recommended treatments for depression are both psychotherapy and pharmacotherapy.[5,6]

CASE RESOLUTION

Months after seeing Mrs. Smith and recommending that she seek care for herself, you see her in the hospital. She thanks you for guiding her to see a health care provider. She is now seeing a psychiatrist and a therapist, who are both valuable in helping her transition back to her previous life. She is now again participating in her church community and family events. She tells you that she is thinking of downsizing and moving closer to her adult children. She is looking forward to seeing her children and grandchildren. She was sorry she cannot chat with you for longer during her visit because she has to go pick up her granddaughter from day care.

- Grief is a normal response to loss, but complicated grief is not.
- Complicated grief will disrupt normal function.
- Some of the risk factors include past history of abuse or neglect, female gender, weak social or spiritual support, short duration of diagnosis to death, and previous diagnosis of depression.
- Identifying and addressing complicated grief in its early stages can prevent progression into clinically significant depression.
- Reducing the frequency of reminders of the passing of their loved ones is recommended to facilitate resuming previous activities.
- Facilitation of expression and processing of grief will decrease the risk of complicated grief. This includes honest and unguarded discussions of prognosis and treatment goals.
- If complicated grief is identified as resulting in depression, it should be treated aggressively.

References

1. Tyrrell P, Harberger S, Schoo C, Siddiqui W. *Kubler-Ross stages of dying and subsequent models of grief*. In *StatPearls*. StatPearls Publishing; 2022.
2. Battle DE. Diagnostic and Statistical Manual of Mental Disorders (DSM). *Codas*. 2013;25(2):191–192.
3. Mason TM, Tofthagen CS, Buck HG. Complicated grief: Risk factors, protective factors, and interventions. *J Soc Work End Life Palliat Care*. 2020;16(2):151–174.
4. Allen JY, Haley WE, Small BJ, Schonwetter RS, McMillan SC. Bereavement among hospice caregivers of cancer patients one year following loss: Predictors of grief, complicated grief, and symptoms of depression. *J Palliat Med*. 2013;16(7):745–751.
5. Zaider T, Kissane D. The assessment and management of family distress during palliative care. *Curr Opin Support Palliat Care*. 2009;3(1):67–71.
6. Simon NM. Treating complicated grief. *JAMA*. 2013;310(4):416–423.

Further Reading

Berger A, O'Neill JF. *Principles and Practice of Palliative Care and Support Oncology*. Wolters Kluwer; 2021.

PART III

Dilemmas Related to Health Care Professionals

15 Moral Distress by Staff: My Patient Is Suffering and "We Can't Keep Torturing Them"

Anthony Eidelman and Regina M. Fink

A 66-year-old retired physician was transferred to the intensive care unit (ICU) from inpatient oncology. Eighteen months previously, he was treated with chemo and radiation therapy for stage 4 diffuse large B cell lymphoma with bulky mediastinal disease. Although he had a complete response, lymphoma reoccurrence was confirmed by biopsy. His medical oncologist offered intensive salvage chemotherapy followed by autologous bone marrow transplantation (BMT). Post-transplant, he developed sepsis and was on a ventilator with multi-organ failure. His wife remained optimistic, hoping for a miracle.

ICU care team (nurses, advance practice providers, and house staff) felt sadness, frustration, and emotional exhaustion. They had difficulty coping with his worsening condition, often discussing what they would do. The BMT team rounded daily, providing its view that "we need for this pancytopenia to resolve so he can get better." An ICU intensivist consulted palliative care to foster communication and help with symptoms. Aggressive treatment continued with no palliative/end-of-life care discussion.

What do you do now?

DISCUSSION

Increasingly, health care providers face challenging demands on their ability to provide adequate care for patients because of time constraints and available resources.[1] *Burnout* has been defined as a mismatch between demands and resources—a state of chronic stress that leads to exhaustion, depersonalization, and lack of accomplishment.[2] In contrast, *moral distress* is an emotional anguish that occurs when an individual believes they are compromising their integrity by being compelled to act in a manner contrary to their moral values. In other words, the clinician knows the ethically correct course of action, but because of circumstances out of their control, they are constrained from doing what they believe is right.[3,4]

Some advocate broadening the definition of moral distress to encompass the psychological distress experienced by a health care professional due to moral uncertainty, conflict, or dilemma.[5] The term *moral injury* is about more than shortfalls of resources and time, and it extends to untenable and unsustainable situations.[3-5] When providers encounter moral uncertainty or are compelled to act in a manner contrary to their moral values, the dissonance between what they can do and should do often weighs heavily. The consequences of unresolved moral distress include diminished provider mental health, impaired resilience, decreased capacity to be compassionate, withdrawal from patients, compromised quality of care, and staff turnover.[4,6] Moral distress is positively correlated with burnout and compassion fatigue, and it may be an underlying precedent to these undesirable outcomes.[6] Moral distress is a potential concern for medical providers regardless of discipline and health care setting. As our case depicts, factors predisposing to moral distress include attending to patients at the end of life, proximity to suffering, and moral doubts regarding care.[4] Moral distress is prevalent in palliative care professionals perhaps related to continuously caring for patients with serious illness and the responsibility to facilitate complicated decisions that often rely on personal discretion and individual values, including those related to the life–death process, artificial support, and relief of suffering.[4]

There have been substantial efforts to develop meaningful strategies to mitigate or, where possible, preempt the experience of moral distress.[7-11] Proposed interventions include reflective practice, cultivating moral resilience, fostering collaborative relationships, effective communication, implementation of educational programs, and improving personal psychological empowerment. Enhancing moral resilience has been proposed as a coping strategy to enable providers to navigate ethically complex situations.[10,11] Developing internal strategies, mindfulness, and self-regulation can help health care professionals respond positively to moral adversity. Although these approaches offer promising direction, further research is necessary to determine the effectiveness of these interventions.[7–9] Currently, no single intervention has been found to reliably mitigate the detrimental effects of moral distress.[7–9] It is likely that future effective strategies to ameliorate moral distress will be multifaceted and address the interrelated dynamics among patients, families, health care providers, and health care organizations. Moral distress is often experienced by providers caring for patients at end of life, when there is uncertainty regarding continuing aggressive care or focusing on comfort and symptom relief. Our case demonstrates that poor communication either among the provider team members or between clinicians and patients with serious illness may be the root cause of moral distress.[4] It is essential to have well-articulated discussions with patients, family caregivers, and their surrogates regarding personal goals, values, and preferences. It is also preferable to begin these conversations early in the illness rather than waiting until crisis or death is imminent. Moral distress may be mitigated through proficient communication and mutually shared decision-making that respects both patient and clinician values. Moral distress is a complex issue that most likely cannot be completely eradicated. However, recognition of moral distress in oneself or colleagues could be viewed a "warning sign" and an indicator of potential ethical concerns that could prompt analysis and intervention.

CASE RESOLUTION

The ICU attending requested a formal palliative care consultation. The palliative care physician communicated with the other medical specialists to obtain consensus regarding prognosis, treatments options, and other relevant issues. A structured family meeting was conducted by the interdisciplinary palliative care team to assess illness understanding, communicate prognosis, and inquire about personal values and preferences. Specific goals of care were formulated using a shared decision-making approach. After taking time to reflect on options, the patient and his wife eventually opt for measures to prolong life even though this would result in ongoing disability and potential suffering. There was clear communication among all parties, including the entire health care team and nursing staff, with respect to goals, values, and reasons for treatment decisions. A debriefing session was facilitated by the palliative care team in the ICU for open conversation, analysis, and support. It was discussed that in health care, inevitably there are circumstances that are out of our control. Patients and their families have autonomy to make care decisions that may contravene our personal beliefs. Nevertheless, it is important to practice self-care and cultivate moral resilience so as not to bear the burden of moral distress.

KEY POINTS TO REMEMBER

- Moral distress is a particular form of moral suffering that is associated with detrimental outcomes, including compromised quality of patient care, impaired provider well-being, and organizational challenges.
- Moral distress affects health professionals across various disciplines and settings. Palliative care providers often experience moral distress, especially as ethical dilemmas abound and there is responsibility to facilitate complicated care decisions.
- It is paramount that palliative care professionals have familiarity with moral distress in order to support themselves and their colleagues and also to implement systems-level interventions.
- Moral distress is often associated with poor communication among providers, patients, family caregivers, or their surrogates.
- There are few proven effective interventions for mitigating the effects of moral distress.
- On an individual level, cultivating moral resilience has been proposed as a coping strategy to support clinicians who experience ethically complex situations.

• It is likely that future effective interventions will be multidimensional and address the complex root causes of moral distress.

References

1. National Academy of Medicine. *National plan for health workforce well-being.* National Academies Press; 2022. https://doi.org/10.17226/26744
2. Rotenstein LS, Torre M, Ramos MA, et al. Prevalence of burnout among physicians: A systematic review. *JAMA.* 2018;320(11):1131–1150.
3. Morley G, Ives J, Bradbury-Jones C, Irvine F. What is "moral distress"? A narrative synthesis of the literature. *Nurs Ethics.* 2019;26(3):646–662.
4. Maffoni M, Argentero P, Giorgil, Hynes J, Giardini A. Healthcare professionals' moral distress in adult palliative care: A systematic review. *BMJ Support Palliat Care.* 2019;9(3):245–254.
5. Fourie C. Who is experiencing what kind of moral distress? Distinctions for moving from a narrow to a broad definition of moral distress. *AMA J Ethics.* 2017;19(6):578–584.
6. McAndrew NS, Leske J, Schroeter K. Moral distress in critical care nursing: The state of the science. *Nurs Ethics.* 2018;25(5):552–570.
7. Imbulana DI, Davis PG, Prentice TM. Interventions to reduce moral distress in clinicians working in intensive care: A systematic review. *Intensive Crit Care Nurs.* 2021;66:103092.
8. Morley G, Field R, Horsburgh CC, Burchill C. Interventions to mitigate moral distress: A systematic review of the literature. *Int J Nurs Stud.* 2021;121:103984.
9. Amos VK, Epstein E. Moral distress interventions: An integrative literature review. *Nurs Ethics.* 2022;29(3):582–607.
10. Heinze KE, Hanson G, Holtz H, Swoboda SM, Rushton CH. Measuring health care interprofessionals' moral resilience: Validation of the Rushton Moral Resilience Scale. *J Palliat Med.* 2021;24(6):865–872.
11. Rushton CH, Schoonover-Shoffner K, Kennedy MS. Executive summary: Transforming moral distress into moral resilience in nursing. *Am J Nurs.* 2017;117(2):52–56.

16 Work–Nonwork Life Fit: Tensions for Health Care Clinicians

Emily P. Guinee, M. Jennifer Cheng,
Angela K. M. Lipshutz, and
Deborah J. Snyder

You are a resident in internal medicine and a parent of two young children. Your partner is deployed overseas, and you do not have close friends or relatives in the area. In the morning, you have to drop off the kids and are sometimes late to morning conference. In the afternoon, you are in a rush to give sign out to your co-residents to make it to day care on time for pick up. You sometimes sense that your co-residents and faculty are frustrated with you. You feel reluctant to share with your co-residents because they probably have their own stresses. You feel reluctant to share with faculty your struggles because you want to appear competent and do not want this to affect your evaluations. You end up spending hours each night finishing clinic notes and preparing for journal club, talks, and projects. You feel guilty and alone. You want to be a good doctor and a good parent, but work–life balance feels unachievable.

What do you do now?

Trainees often give up control of their lives during the time-consuming period that is residency. Often, you are burning the candle at both ends, which may lead to burnout and negative consequences to patients, health care systems, you, and your family. Over your career, you will encounter challenges in how to best prioritize your finite energy and integrate your personal life with your professional life. Taking the time to understand and manage these challenges is an important goal for all physicians and health care professionals to consider.

As a palliative care clinician, you are trained to acknowledge the humanity of your patients. You must also acknowledge your own humanity, which includes recognizing that you cannot be all things to all people all the time. You are not inexhaustible. Something has got to give. It is important to understand how efforts can be made personally, professionally, and organizationally to support a more achievable "work–nonwork life fit." Although many know the verbiage "work–life balance," we believe this term connotes that life stops when you are at work and work stops when you are living. As a clinician, you know this not to be true. "Balance" also suggests a polarity between work and life. As long as we believe this polarity to exist, we will always encounter the conflict that accompanies polarity.[1] Thus, we posit that clinicians and workplaces can endeavor to fit work and nonwork life together. Palliative care is an interdisciplinary specialty that relies on providers with various expertise. This chapter focuses on the case of a physician resident, but its message applies to all health care providers.

Issues of trainee burnout and work–nonwork life fit struggles are highly prevalent, and increasing, in graduate medical education. Studies on burnout and satisfaction with work–life integration showed that 62.8% of physicians reported at least one major symptom of burnout in 2021, compared to 38.2% in 2020.[2] A similar trend was seen for work–life integration, such that satisfaction with work–life integration decreased from 46.1% to 30.2% between 2020 and 2021.[2] These well-being concerns exist for all types of health care professionals within palliative care.[3,4] One-fourth of palliative care nurses report at least one symptom of burnout, and burnout prevalence does not seem to vary significantly between nurses and physicians providing palliative care.[4,5] The medical field must acknowledge that individuals have challenges of varying intensities, at different times of life, and that everyone should play a role in establishing a culture of caring.

Indeed, there has been a renewed emphasis on clinician well-being recently, prompting a slow but consistent culture shift in medicine. Consider, for example, the Accreditation Council for Graduate Medical Education 2017 guidelines, which established a requirement around physician well-being, or the establishment of the Well-Being Initiative from the American Nurses Foundation.[6,7] In 2016, leaders at Stanford University presented the Stanford Model of Professional Fulfillment, which emphasized that achieving professional fulfillment and mitigating against burnout required a focus on not only internal (personal) drivers of burnout but also external ones related to organizational structure and culture. The model identifies three domains: the culture of wellness, efficiency of practice, and personal resilience.[8] Many health care systems have integrated components of personal resilience into their workplace, for example, by encouraging mindfulness-based practice, yoga, exercise, sleep mitigation, and managing mental health issues. In addition, some health care systems have promoted a culture of wellness by engaging leadership in wellness initiatives and even creating a Chief Wellness Officer position.[9,10] Implementation of structural changes to improve efficiency of practice, however, has been slower to take off. Also, some expectations that have historically been embedded in the practice of medicine, such as "fake it until you make it" or not complaining, are more difficult to refashion.

You are now armed with the knowledge that we hope makes you feel more empowered, less alone, and aware of the data. With this understanding, you can take actions to address internal and external drivers that perturb your work–nonwork life fit. The first step is to look inward to examine your internal distress. People have different tolerances for distress. Likewise, individuals have distinct styles for coping with stress and discomfort. Reflect on your personal style, and gauge where you are on your own distress thermometer; try to be cognizant of your threshold from stretched to stressed. Then, be introspective and ask yourself: What is driving my burnout? As you consider the abundance of familial, personal, and professional responsibilities you hold, be conscious of your cognitive distortions, such as the erroneous idea that one can handle anything that is thrown one's way. In this case, the challenge is related to being a single parent who has the sole responsibility for managing children in the context of a demanding medical career. Separate each step, for example, coming in late to a didactic, leaving early and needing to transition with peers, and taking work home after hours. Although some changes can be made internally and in the non-work domains of life, much of the stress comes from the job demands that are placed on health care professionals.

Now begin to consider the workplace shifts that can be made. Although practicing medicine is a self-sacrificial profession, you must advocate for your own well-being throughout your training and career. This is true for all health care professionals because the risks are simply too high if you do not pause and reflect on what is missing in professional spaces. In this moment of reflection, think about what your goals are. Throughout this process, reflect on what you can, cannot, and wish you could control. Do your part in identifying solutions to your challenges, in both work and non-work life, and share these potential solutions as you open up to colleagues. Do you need time for replenishment? Do you need more support? Do you need to make a specific request, such as formally shifting your schedule? Understand what you are asking for, then consider who you should ask. Who, at work, do you feel most safe with? This might be a peer, a trusted faculty member, or your supervisor. Or rather, might there be like-minded, like-experienced colleagues? Identify this person or affinity group and think about if they can offer you what you need in the given moment. Some people can provide direct support, whereas others can help brainstorm creative solutions. Consider practicing these conversations outside of the work setting. If you are hesitant to have these conversations with colleagues, remember that health care is a team sport. Interdependence and trust with peers are essential for both effectively and safely caring for patients and establishing boundaries. If you are in academic medicine and your responsibilities extend beyond patient care, think about the other tasks you must manage. Although your requests might put demands on others, starting these discussions is the first step in reducing your own sense of isolation, and it may even reduce feelings of isolation in others. You can begin to promote a culture of openness, vulnerability, and well-being through these conversations. Solutions, sometimes even unexpected ones, can come through having open conversations.

After commencing workplace conversations, equip yourself with an understanding of potential workplace solutions that already exist. Are there resources available in your environment that may help address the challenges you are facing? In the case of our vignette, for example, perhaps there are onsite childcare options, librarian support for literature reviews, or shortcuts in the electronic medical record that increase efficiency.

As you identify and implement solutions that improve your work–nonwork life fit, you may want to consider what organizational changes can be instituted to support work–nonwork life fit at your institution more generally. For example, you can investigate whether your program has a formal way of tracking well-being and work–nonwork life fit among trainees. If it does not exist, consider advocating for it in partnership with colleagues, mentors, or graduate medical education (GME) leaders. Tracking well-being with surveys such as the Well-Being Index from the Mayo Clinic or the Professional Quality of Life Measure would allow program directors, supervisors, and other leaders to understand clinician well-being and emphasize the need for further investment in interventions that both proactively prevent burnout and reactively respond to high levels of distress.[11,12] Or, you may choose a quality improvement project topic that focuses on improving workflows or identifying key drivers of burnout within your program or department. Examining well-being systematically may uncover challenges that clinicians within your department unknowingly share and allow for program-level or even institution-level interventions.

It is our hope that now you have the knowledge of national policies that underscore the importance of your own well-being, of various questions that you can reflect on within yourself, and of questions to ask of your institution about well-being resources and the potential for systematic change. We have summarized our top 10 suggestions for reflection and action in Box 16.1. Finally, remember that sometimes features of burnout can present similarly to clinical mental health symptoms. If symptoms begin to impact functioning at work or in nonwork life, consider reaching out to professional services. You can talk to professionals at your employee assistance program, 24/7 crisis lines, or mental health clinicians. If you are comfortable asking leadership, your program director could also direct you to services. Consider involving the office of the ombudsman or the GME office if challenges persist or if you believe there is a toxic work environment that prevents you from speaking up. Author and philosopher Alain de Botton says, "There is no such thing as work–life balance. Everything

BOX 16.1 **Top 10 Tips for Enhancing Work–Nonwork Life Fit**

1. Arm yourself with knowledge about national governing bodies that have standards regarding clinician well-being.
2. Identify your threshold from stretched to stressed.
3. Give yourself grace and remember that you are not inexhaustible.
4. Identify what can and cannot be changed at work and in your nonwork life.
5. Identify existing resources and solutions before making workplace requests.
6. Talk to trusted colleagues, and remember that health care is a team endeavor.
7. In partnership with colleagues, advocate for organizational well-being initiatives.
8. Use your quality improvement project to evaluate well-being to help normalize this topic.
9. Continuously engage in introspection.
10. If your symptoms of burnout impact your functioning at work and/or in nonwork life, consider reaching out to a mental health professional.

worth fighting for unbalances your life." Remember that although you might not achieve perfect balance, your own well-being is very much worth fighting for.

KEY POINTS TO REMEMBER

- Clinician burnout is common in health care and has been increasing in recent years.
- We suggest conceptualizing well-being as fitting together work and nonwork life, rather than focusing on achieving a "balance." Work–nonwork life fit avoids the polarity of "balance" and acknowledges that work is life and the proportional importance of work and nonwork life may shift over time.
- The Stanford Model of Professional Fulfillment identifies three domains: culture of wellness, efficiency of practice, and personal resilience. This model is applicable across disciplines

and can be readily considered when tackling issues related to burnout and well-being.

- In addressing your own challenges with work–nonwork fit, we suggest introspection, discussion with a trusted colleague, identification of existing institutional resources, and exploration of opportunities to address well-being at a systems level.
- Remember that health care is a team endeavor in which interdependence and trusting others are essential for patient care. These traits are also essential for establishing work–nonwork life fit and appropriate boundaries when possible.
- If symptoms are moving from burnout to symptoms impacting functioning at work and in nonwork life, consider reaching out to mental health professional services and talking directly with your program director or supervisor.

References

1. Schwingshackl A. The fallacy of chasing after work–life balance. *Front Pediatr.* 2014;2:26. doi:10.3389/fped.2014.00026
2. Shanafelt TD, West CP, Dyrbye LN, et al. Changes in burnout and satisfaction with work–life integration in physicians during the first 2 years of the COVID-19 pandemic. *Mayo Clin Proc.* 2022;97(12):2248–2258. doi:10.1016/j.mayocp.2022.09.002
3. Harrison KL, Dzeng E, Ritchie CS, et al. Addressing palliative care clinician burnout in organizations: A workforce necessity, an ethical imperative. *J Pain Symptom Manage.* 2017;53(6):1091–1096. doi:10.1016/j.jpainsymman.2017.01.007
4. Gómez-Urquiza JL, Albendín-García L, Velando-Soriano A, et al. Burnout in palliative care nurses, prevalence and risk factors: A systematic review with meta-analysis. *Int J Environ Res Public Health.* 2020;17(20):7672. doi:10.3390/ijerph17207672
5. Dijxhoorn A-FQ, Brom L, van der Linden YM, Leget C, Raijmakers NJH. Prevalence of burnout in healthcare professionals providing palliative care and the effect of interventions to reduce symptoms: A systematic literature review. *Palliat Med.* 2021;35(1):6–26. doi:10.1177/0269216320956825
6. Accreditation Council for Graduate Medical Education. ACGME common program requirements (fellowship). 2017. https://www.acgme.org/globalassets/pfassets/programrequirements/cprfellowship_2023v3.pdf
7. American Nurses Foundation. American Nurses Foundation launches national well-being initiative for nurses. May 19, 2020. https://www.nursingworld.org/

news/news-releases/2020/american-nurses-foundation-launches-national-well-being-initiative-for-nurses

8. Bohman B, Dyrbye L, Sinsky CA, et al. Physician well-being: The reciprocity of practice efficiency, culture of wellness, and personal resilience. *NEJM Catalyst.* August 7, 2017;

9. Ripp J, Shanafelt T. The health care chief wellness officer: What the role is and is not. *Acad Med.* 2020;95(9):1354–1358. doi:10.1097/acm.0000000000003433

10. Shanafelt T, Trockel M, Rodriguez A, Logan D. Wellness-centered leadership: Equipping health care leaders to cultivate physician well-being and professional fulfillment. *Acad Med.* 2021;96(5):641–651.

11. Dyrbye LN, Satele D, Sloan J, Shanafelt TD. Utility of a brief screening tool to identify physicians in distress. *J Gen Intern Med.* 2013;28(3):421–427. doi:10.1007/s11606-012-2252-9

12. Stamm BH. Professional Quality of Life: Compassion Satisfaction and Fatigue Version 5 (ProQOL). http://proqol.org

Burnout and Resilience

Jennifer Winegarden and
Ylisabyth Bradshaw

As an unhoused, severe alcoholic, Ricky's case challenged the entire hospital system. Worsening organ failure was documented each time a concerned bystander found him unresponsive in the street and called 911. Without an advance directive or power of attorney, each hospitalization included increasingly complex life-saving treatment. Now he lay unresponsive and ventilated in septic shock, with hepatorenal syndrome and anoxic brain injury. His closest friend and the medical team were in the process of agreeing to stop all life-saving treatments when his estranged children arrived. After the court awarded them emergency custody, they asked for a tracheotomy, feeding tube, and any aggressive measure that could prolong his life. As the senior team leader of the palliative department, you are scheduled to leave on vacation. Your young team struggles through the stressors, and despite your family's need for your attention, you find you cannot stop reading the notes and texting your colleagues.

What do you do now?

DISCUSSION

Of the many desirable attributes a physician may develop, perhaps none is as worthy as perseverance. This idea, based on a concept of endurance, describes the character that progresses from "strength to strength" despite facing frequent trials. This type of fortitude arises from the actions of those who carry another's burden. An example can be drawn from the life of Dr. William Worrall Mayo, whose practice grew from the destruction of a tornado in 1883 in his rural town in Minnesota. Within a community facing poverty and need, he and his sons, William and Charles, developed a thriving practice. Although often paid in chickens or vegetables, the Doctors Mayo developed a professional heartiness that facilitated medical advancements. This type of practice resourcefulness arises not from lack of struggle but, rather, from overcoming significant stressors while maintaining selfless dedication and resilience.

The complexity, however, of American medical practice has greatly increased and so have its challenges and frustrations. The first discussion of clinician burnout was published by psychologist Herbert Freudenberger in 1974. He noted its effect in professionals and volunteer staff who were intensely dedicated and became overextended, internally driven to serve and externally motivated by the needs and suffering of their patients.[1] Consistent with earlier work in the study of air traffic controllers,[2] Freudenberger's findings showed that professionals who were most dedicated to the organizational mission, committed to service excellence, and most altruistic were often at the greatest risk of professional burnout.[1] Although not exclusive to medicine, this sense of dedication is rooted in our profession, which has been continually called upon to rise above instincts of self-preservation to care for those who face significant suffering. So clearly has this been the sine qua non of the character of a physician that many seeking an altruistic career are drawn to its practice, including Dame Cicely Saunders, Albert Schweitzer, and Oliver Wendell Holmes.

During the past several decades, the literature has documented increased physician burnout and has expanded to also measure work engagement and explore clinician resilience. The COVID era brought increased self-reporting of physician burnout, and in 2022 the burnout among physicians reached an all-time-high of 47%,[3] with 63% of physicians reporting experiencing at least one symptom of burnout, an increase of 44% in 4 years.[4]

In the 11th revision of the *International Classification of Diseases*, the World Health Organization (WHO) added further detail, defining burnout as a

> syndrome conceptualized as resulting from chronic workplace stress that has not been successfully managed [that] . . . is characterized by three dimensions: 1) feelings of energy depletion or exhaustion; 2) increased mental distance from one's job, or feelings of negativism or cynicism related to one's job; and 3) reduced professional efficacy.[5,6]

The WHO explicitly notes that burnout occurs in an occupational context and is not applied to other life experiences; burnout is not defined as a mental health condition.

Burnout has long been associated with people-oriented, caring professions that expect a selfless ethos and a focus on service to others in working conditions with high demands, limited resources, and long hours. The following are three important predispositions to developing burnout:

1. A commitment to excellence, also seen as altruism, compassion (as in compassion fatigue), and an elevated level of dedication with internal drive for ideals.
2. Continued stressors with consistent levels of difficulty, frequent changes, loss of control in areas of job domain, and external pressure or needs to be overcommitted.
3. Given the conditions described in 1 and 2, the clinician becomes enmeshed in the current environment and unable to become rejuvenated. Clinical practice has become a routine with a sense that no progress can be made.

It is not difficult to recall a physician who began their practice as a compassionate and driven individual who now appears cynical or calculating in the workplace. Such changes indicate a poor response to continual stress and a withdrawal from the traits once viewed as ideal. In fact, such a physician may now cynically view others who have compassion and empathetic capacity as inexperienced or naive. To the contrary, the compassionate physician never views themself so removed from the suffering and stressors of illness that they lose their sympathy or empathy.

The causal linkages in developing burnout are still being studied. Conceptually, burnout was initially considered to occur in sequential stages, with exhaustion due to high work demands occurring first, leading to depersonalization or cynicism and, finally, to a decreased sense of personal accomplishment with feelings of inadequacy and failure.[7] More recent developmental burnout models focus on the imbalance between work demands and available resources. These models can be restricted to the perspective of the individual, but more usefully can be applied at the organizational level.[8] One such framework is the Areas of Worklife model that identifies key domains for person–job mismatches to occur with higher risk of burnout or concordant matches to occur with greater probability of substantial work engagement.[9] These domains are workload, control, reward, community, fairness, and values.

Finding solutions to these alarming trends has not been straightforward. Programs aimed at developing and sustaining clinician resilience have provided greater awareness of practical actions that individuals can take while also stimulating research. Epstein and Krasner, in a commentary from 2013, provided the following definition: "Resilience is the capacity to respond to stress in a healthy way such that goals are achieved at minimal psychological and physical cost; resilient individuals 'bounce back' after challenges while also growing stronger."[10]

Adaptation and the development of resilient and sustainable practice are both the responsibility of each individual physician and a function of the system in which they work. Many hospitals, conferences, and online presentations address avenues for individual resilience training, creating the perception that it is the clinician alone who has the ability to apply and adapt to such education.[11,12] The Surgeon General's advisory on "Addressing Health Worker Burnout"[13] and earlier National Academy of Medicine initiatives[11,14] provide recognition of the importance of organizations and the health care system in preventing physician and other health care worker burnout. Evidence supports greater impact from interventions focused on organizational change than those that are physician-directed.[15] Yet, there is also a shared role of responsibility in the concept of career-long resiliency training. A comprehensive model promotes resiliency training that begins with medical education, continues through training, and is supported throughout all stages of practice, calling for medical school and institutional involvement to sequentially address the "inevitable toll of being a healthcare professional."[12]

Transforming workplace cultures to cultivate and empower staff in participatory management and open communication is an initial step in valuing health care workers. Integrating health and safety, ensuring access to appropriate physical and mental health and substance use needs, prioritizing community and social connection, as well as quality time with patients and colleagues are important.[14] Further significant initiatives for preventing and treating burnout articulated by the Surgeon General are combating bias, racism, and discrimination in the workplace; confronting health misinformation; and addressing health inequities. Resources to meet professional job demands should be available both through the workplace and through one's own personal capacity. Neither source is sufficient by itself.

An insightful study of more than 200 physicians from varied disciplines provides a typology for types of resilience strategies used by experienced successful physicians.[16] Researchers interviewed these physicians and classified their strategies into three categories. (1) Work-related sources of gratification comprised the first category; these included direct satisfaction from the doctor–patient relationship as well as fulfillment from intervening and changing the disease course through efficacious medical care. (2) Address practices and routine changes, such as limiting working hours, cultivating leisure time and social relationships, proactively engaging with the limitations and uncertainties in medical practice, personal reflection, and spiritual practices. (3) Create resilience strategies; including useful attitudes and mindsets characterized as acceptance and realism, self-awareness and reflexivity, active engagement with the downsides of medicine, recognizing when change was necessary, and appreciating the good things.

Being aware of one's own level of stress, and how to engage the needed coping mechanisms, is the beginning of this type of self-management. Change comes once previously compensated environmental responses become those of adaptive stress management, leading to a freedom in accepting continual challenges and thriving in (and despite) the stressors. Developing a practice of resilience meets an ultimate realization through personal acceptance of risks and the ability to change. To fully address the natural stressors of medical practice and the individual responsibility to maintain professional health, physicians must maintain a level of commitment to the following:

1. Mindfulness—a practice of being in the moment with awareness to accept or release situations that are out of one's control, even in the past or future
2. Self-monitoring—the ability to monitor one's own boundaries, emotional involvement or professional pride, and/or seek out the opinions of colleagues
3. Limit-setting—keeping at once both emotional appropriateness and maintaining a professional distance[17]

Although a physician's resilience can be affected by institutional situations outside of their control, there are many individual practices and characteristics that help dictate a physician's healthy lifestyle. Such practices may have been developed during the undergraduate or medical school years and can be relied on much later in life. These include stimulating conferences or academic pursuits, time spent in meditation and spiritual or physical enrichment, family gatherings, and restful vacations. Physicians new to practice may be less likely to maintain firm boundaries, carrying with them an increased risk of burnout.[14] Therefore, early in one's career, it is critical to develop habits that build rejuvenation and resilience.

Professional resilience maintains that while improved practice parameters are being sought, one's personal response is to avoid negative attitudes and other emotional reactions to stress. Control of responses within individual experiences can prevent the chronic engagement of such. Continued self-care with healthy emotional and physical habits and intentional cognitive and emotional flexibility are key. Professional fulfillment can still be attained when progress toward a culture of wellness, efficiency of practice, and personal resilience is achieved.[18]

When each of the factors leading to burnout can be addressed individually, and progress made toward practice realization, resiliency skills and healthy boundaries can develop.[19] "Boundaries in clinical medicine are the limitations we place around the emotional and physical relationships between patients and providers and between medical colleagues."[17(p.417)] When a clinician is unsure of whether their relationships are professional, the following question should be asked of themself and opinions sought by other trusted colleagues. "Is my role adhering to that of my job description with an appropriate level of emotional involvement?" For those who struggle with overresponsibility, a backup question may be, "Do I believe that I am the only team member who can see the patient [due to a self-assigned role of importance] or am I simply the most appropriate clinician to provide care today?" Keeping balance in both patient and collegial relationships leads to healthy work and home relationships, prevents burnout, and can greatly aid the development of resilience.

CASE RESOLUTION

Following several days of increased family tensions, this senior clinician's self-reflection and supportive challenging queries from her spouse brought greater self-awareness. She realized she was over-enmeshed and nearing burnout levels at work, and it was having a negative effect on her family relationships. With the distance from work and opportunity for reflection, she recognized that in addition to her own boundary-setting failures, there were structural and organizational weaknesses within her institution. She realized that she did not have to be a solo leader. The young palliative team needed the support and engagement of an associate team leader. Inquiries led to a physician from the family medicine department with hospice and palliative experience who was willing to step in when needed. This organizational commitment led to additional support and an alternate point of contact.

When discussing the situation with another trusted colleague, the two physicians decided to hold each other accountable for resilience-based activities and provide a much-needed safe place for collegial support.

Within the palliative department, group education around resiliency topics and a "resilience-building activity" were completed. With this success, the group planned for further resilience discussions in future meetings as well as one team-enriching group event per quarter.

When discussing this situation with her husband, the physician discovered new insight into what made this situation so difficult to let go of. Together, they worked to schedule couple and family times away from home on a regular basis.

- The complexity and inherent demands of a palliative medicine career require physicians to have a heightened sense of self-awareness.
- The most altruistic practitioners are at the greatest risk of burn-out.
- Resilience, or professional heartiness, occurs when physicians rise above workplace stressors while growing stronger.
- The most effective resiliency training involves workplace initiatives with clinician's growth toward adaptive stress management.

References

1. Freudenberger HJ. Staff burn-out. *J Soc Issues*. 1974;30(1):159–165. https://doi.org/10.1111/j.1540-4560.1974.tb00706.x
2. Samra R. Brief history of burnout. *BMJ*. 2018;363:k5268. https://www.bmj.com/content/363/bmj.k5268.full
3. iPRO. The state of physician burnout in 2022. March 18, 2022. https://healthcare.ipro-inc.com/blog/the-state-of-physician-burnout-in-2022/
4. Tait D, Shanafelt MD, West CP, Lotte N. Changes in burnout and satisfaction with work–life integration in physicians during the first 2 years of the COVID-19 pandemic. *Mayo Clin Proc*. 2022;97(12):2248–2258 https://mayoclinic.pure.elsevier.com/en/publications/changes-in-burnout-and-satisfaction-with-work-life-balance-in-phy
5. World Health Organization. Burn-out an "occupational phenomenon": International Classification of Diseases (ICD-11). May 28, 2019. https://www.who.int/news/item/28-05-2019-burn-out-an-occupational-phenomenon-international-classification-of-diseases
6. World Health Organization. ICD-11 for mortality and morbidity statistics. 2022. https://icd.who.int/browse11/l-m/en#/http://id.who.int/icd/entity/129180281
7. Maslach C, Leiter MP. Understanding the burnout experience: Recent research and its implications for psychiatry. *World Psychiatry*. 2016;15(2):103–11. doi:10.1002/wps.20311
8. Shanafelt TD, Dyrbye LN, West CP. Addressing physician burnout: The way forward. *JAMA*. 2017;317(9):901–902. doi:10.1001/jama.2017.0076
9. Leiter MP, Maslach C. Areas of worklife: A structured approach to organizational predictors of job burnout. In: Perrewé PL, Ganster DC, eds. *Emotional and Physiological Processes and Positive Intervention Strategies*. Elsevier; 2004:91–134.

10. Epstein RM, Krasner MS. Physician resilience: What it means, why it matters, and how to promote it. *Acad Med*. 2013;88(3):301–303. doi:10.1097/ACM.0b013e318280cff0

11. National Academy of Medicine. Taking action against clinician burnout: A systems approach to professional well being report release event. October 23, 2019. https://nam.edu/event/taking-action-against-clinician-burnout-a-systems-approach-to-professional-well-being-report-release-event

12. Cordova MJ, Gimmler CE, Osterberg LG. Foster well-being throughout the career trajectory: A developmental model of physician resilience training. *Mayo Clin Proc*. 2020;95(12):2719–2733. https://www.mayoclinicproceedings.org/article/S0025-6196(20)30469-9/fulltext

13. Office of the Surgeon General. Addressing health worker burnout: The U.S. Surgeon General's advisory on building a thriving health workforce. May 2022. https://www.hhs.gov/sites/default/files/health-worker-wellbeing-advisory.pdf

14. Dyrbye LN, TD Shanafelt TD, Sinsky CA, et al. Burnout among health care professionals: A call to explore and address this underrecognized threat to safe, high-quality care. National Academy of Medicine. July 5, 2017. https://nam.edu/wp-content/uploads/2017/07/Burnout-Among-Health-Care-Professionals-A-Call-to-Explore-and-Address-This-Underrecognized-Threat.pdf

15. Panagioti M, Panagopoulou E, Bower P, et al. Controlled interventions to reduce burnout in physicians: A systematic review and meta-analysis. *JAMA Intern Med*. 2017;177(2):195–205.

16. Zwack J, Schweitzer J. If every fifth physician is affected by burnout, what about the other four? Resilience strategies of experienced physicians. *Acad Med*. 2013;88(3):382–389. doi:10.1097/ACM.0b013e318281696b

17. Lawton C, Lawton AJ, Stephens E., et al. Where do we draw the line? Navigating personal and professional boundary challenges in palliative care. *J Pain Symptom Manage*. 2019;57(2):417.

18. Stanford Medicine. The Stanford Model of Professional Fulfillment. 2024. https://wellmd.stanford.edu/about/model-external.html

19. Back AL, Steinhauser KE, Kamal AH, Jackson VA. Building resilience for palliative care clinicians: An approach to burnout prevention based on individual skills and workplace factors. *J Pain Symptom Manage*. 2016;52(2):284–291. https://doi.org/10.1016/j.jpainsymman.2016.02.002

18 Planning and Facing Retirement

Daniel B. Carr and Stephen Gullo

Dr. K is a male palliative care physician in his late 70s. He has worked in this field for more than four decades. He is an active member of both local and national professional associations and societies, and he has served on corporate boards. He is a professor in a medical school and has an interest in theology that started with warm memories of religious holidays as a child. Furthermore, he is interested in astronomy and enjoys an occasional round of golf. He has a positive relationship with his children, but their secular careers and geographical distance separate them from their aging father.

The doctor has a dwindling number of close friends as age, illness, and death have reduced his circle. He has few friends outside of his profession. He was recently predeceased by his wife and is in the midst of a life rebuild as he navigates grief, the loss of identity in his immediate family as a husband, and the loss of his couple-based lifestyle. A large part of his identity comes from his work with professional colleagues and projects within the field. He asks you for advice to better navigate these transitions.

What do you do now?

DISCUSSION

When a person's life has centered on their professional activities, a pre-retirement plan is critical as they near and start to think about retirement. Working professionals managing their lives have been busy socially and professionally, and they are often physically active. Their already diversified, balanced lifestyle may offer them lower hurdles to surmount to achieve a happy retirement, but all retirees benefit from creating a flexible yet actionable pre-retirement plan.

Essential for success in coping with life changes is psychological resilience.[1,2] Just as there is physical fitness over which we have control and that can be enhanced by shrewd life decisions, there is psychological fitness. At the core of psychological fitness is psychological resilience—the emotional shock absorber of the human psyche that allows us to respond positively to change and also, when necessary, to loss. Clinicians involved with palliative care navigate the processes of loss and recovery throughout their tenure with their patients and the patients' families and also in their own lives. The loss of family, peers, youth, health, and physical mobility may follow. Weight gain may follow adoption of a more sedentary lifestyle or an increase in unstructured free time and boredom. Activation of resilience tools may also occur: embracing change; learning to live happily in the face of unhappy circumstances; and permission to feel uncomfortable with fluctuating thoughts and feelings such as uncertainty and lack of clarity, anxiety, grief, and hope. Palliative care clinicians can draw upon their experience and expertise in empathetically helping patients, managing patients' expectations and disappointments. Qualities such as patience, determination, stamina, and constant affirmation of progress where present are vital tools to cultivate a positive mindset toward themselves and their own approaching journey of planning for retirement and living out that plan. In many ways, a lifelong career in palliative care is a lifelong preparation for dealing with the challenges that aging and retirement bring. In working with each patient, you taught them the very qualities and tools that we speak of here—tools that nurture adaptation to the future ahead. Life has presented you with the opportunity to apply that wisdom to your own journey.

As you make plans to retire, you may have feelings or episodes of bleakness, isolation, and futility. One of the major lessons co-author Stephen Gullo learned in working with terminally ill patients was witnessing them plead "If only I had a year, I would . . . ." Because we are not guaranteed tomorrow, the important lesson to learn is "do it now." The meticulous and diligent effort prosperous people expend to prepare a financial estate plan needs to be applied to prepare a life plan that includes an early chapter outlining a pre-retirement plan. Hundreds of print- and web-based resources guide and offer wisdom to retirees from perspectives ranging from empirical behavioral science and epidemiology[1-3] to explicitly and traditionally religious[4-6] and somewhere in between.[7]

Pre-retirement planning must include investing sufficient time to develop a social network outside of work, either through the community at large or through religious or professional activities. The Harvard study on happiness, among the longest studies ever undertaken on human happiness, discovered that there is a direct correlation between the quality of your social network and the quality of your life.[3] A similar conclusion was reached regarding general health and longevity in an eight-decade observational study at Stanford.[1] It is crucial for professionals to start planning with their loved ones, colleagues, and mentors—those who are likewise experiencing this journey. In doing so, they may be able to circumvent the depression, anxiety, loss of motivation, or apathy toward life that in turn give rise to negative health habits connected with eating, drinking and other forms of substance abuse disorders, gambling, and other compulsive and addictive behaviors.[8]

We urge all approaching retirement to adopt a "happiness mission"— a sweeping goal that unifies and drives one's actions. Attitude is critical, whether it be when facing retirement or any major life commitment. To achieve happiness, you should not just expect to be happy; you have to expend energy and effort to become happy.

If, as you read this, you feel you lack sufficient psychological resilience and cognitive flexibility, and struggle with issues of rigidity, that does not mean you will not do well in retirement. However, a strong case can be made for pre-retirement counseling, which we recommend if you have reservations about this next chapter of your life. It is also important to see the broader picture of the joys and the personal goals left uncompleted

BOX 18.1 **Variables That May Make Retirement Less Desirable**

- Troubled marriage or home situation
- No hobbies or interests outside of work
- Adjusted work schedule
- Limited social network outside of work
- Limited or no connection to family due to distance or death
- Society's need of your valuable skills
- Losing and finding identity
- Personal vulnerabilities or vices that may surface with unstructured free time
- Pre-existing health and emotional conditions that work masks or distracts
- Depression

because of the demands of your professional life. You now have the time to work on personal goals, including the dreams that remain. Indeed, for many, retirement may even be a happier and more fulfilling period than one's work life has provided up to now.

Personal happiness has been shown to be enhanced by participation in volunteer service, an activity that incites feelings of making a contribution in working for the betterment of a person, community, society, and oneself. The feeling of being needed is part of social attachment that brings deep fulfillment to a person's life. Happiness takes work, and you have to be willing to do the necessary work developing interpersonal and resilience skills and stamina in new, uncomfortable, and even difficult environments. Do not view happiness as something ingested with no labor; rather, view it as a sustained consequence that will be achieved after diligent effort. Happy people understand it is not a given but, rather, something we create for ourselves. It is a process of learning what works and what does not work for your life at different periods (Box 18.1).

CASE RESOLUTION

The patient identified and acknowledged multiple predictors of post-retirement feelings of meaningfulness and worked to harness these in his everyday life:

- Happy family dynamic
- Numerous friends, quality being more important than quantity
- Intellectual and physical challenges to face
- Financial, quality of life, and lifestyle considerations
- Paid or volunteer activity that involves cognitive awareness and community and social involvement
- Before retiring, it is important to estimate the practical likelihood of implementing a social network outside of work through community, religious, or professional activities.
- Because Dr. K found professional work to be gratifying, one of the positive aspects to retirement is the possibility of teaching because the number of professionals in the field of palliative care is inadequate.

SUMMARY

Retirement is a major life step. For some, it is a joyful step; for others, it is hesitant; and for still others, it involves great trepidation. Whatever your step might be, it is important to have a life plan for moving forward into the next chapter.

Much has been lectured and written about this phase of life.[9] After reading and synthesizing this material and your thoughts and feelings on it, imagine that today is your last day of work: What will you live to wake up for, and will it be rewarding?

RECOMMENDATIONS

"Don't retire from . . . retire to."

—Stephen Gullo, PhD

Construct and carry out a pre-retirement plan:

- Join a bereavement support group.
- Reconnect and cultivate interest in environmental, political, or spiritual endeavors to make social connections with people, groups, or organizations.

- Develop new, active sensorimotor skill sets, such as golf, tennis, and pickleball.
- Sign up for a course in a hobby or an interest that appeals to you, and connect with social groups involved in that endeavor.
- Pursue teaching and mentorship for a local university or college or groups such as Big Brothers/Big Sisters. There are few life forces as strong as the feeling of being needed and making a meaningful contribution to the life of another.
- Volunteer as an educator or participate in a field that involves your new interest.
- Plan activities that excite your passions and are life-enhancing, such as travel, intellectual pursuits, and community involvement.
- Construct a health plan with a doctor, health coach, and trainer involving medical checkups, exercise, and diet.
- Deal with losses, not by withdrawing into a world of depression but by reaching out to bereavement support groups or psychologists in person or online.
- Develop deep and meaningful friendships with people of different ages, particularly younger people with whom you can enjoy spending time sharing accountability for your interests and goals.

KEY POINTS TO REMEMBER

- With any major life change, there is a learning curve.
- Certain activities may not be as rewarding as anticipated.
- Even if you have the wrong answer, you do not have to be paralyzed by fear or anxiety; embrace innovation and face new challenges.
- It is part of the emotional process to feel insecurity or anxiety when approaching retirement because it involves changes financially, professionally, and socially. It is a major life step that will bring these emotions to the forefront.
- Willingness to engage in new activities, not as a "have to do" but as a "want to accomplish" list, will increase happiness and longevity.

- Do not just think about the plan—act on it and set deadlines so that it is not "I'll get to it" but, rather, "I've done it."
- Grant yourself permission to feel anxiety, uncertainty, and hesitation during this important life step and major life change.
- Initiate life-enhancing skills—for example, take a course; take up a musical instrument; take voice or creative writing lessons; join social or nature groups; or begin an engaging and intellectual pursuit.
- If you sense major unresolved feelings such as grief or anxiety are getting in the way of effective retiring, consider counseling in terms of positive psychology, not in terms of "something is wrong with me."
- Network with others who have retired and are executing their own plans.
- If you have doubts about your suitability for retirement, take a short leave of absence for 60–90 days to see if retirement suits you.
- Construct a daily schedule with short- and long-term goals and mileposts.

ACKNOWLEDGMENT

We thank Christopher Miller for editorial and research assistance.

References
1. Friedman H, Martin LR. *The Longevity Project: Surprising Discoveries for Health and Long Life from the Landmark Eight-Decade Study*. Penguin; 2011.
2. Levitin, D. *Successful Aging*. Dutton; 2020.
3. Vaillant G. *Aging Well*. Little, Brown Spark; 2002.
4. Moffic E. *The Happiness Prayer: Ancient Jewish Wisdom for the Best Way to Live Today*. Center Street; 2017.
5. Steinsaltz A. *The Essential Talmud*. Basic Books; 2006.
6. Richo D. *The Five Things We Cannot Change . . . and the Happiness We Find by Embracing Them*. Shambhala; 2005.
7. Lamb F. *Meditate Yourself Happy: Change Your Mood Through Daily Meditation*. Hardie Grant Books; 2023.

8. Zullo AR, Danko KJ, Moyo P, et al. Prevention, diagnosis, and management of opioids, opioid misuse, and opioid use disorder in older adults. Technical Brief No. 37. AHRQ Publication No. 21-EHC005. Agency for Healthcare Research and Quality. November 2020.

9. Schulz M, Waldinger R. *The Good Life: Lessons from the World's Longest Scientific Study of Happiness*. Simon & Schuster; 2023.

PART IV

Dilemmas Related to the Health Care System

Balancing Opioid Benefit and Risk for Subacute or Chronic Non-Cancer Pain

Scott A. Strassels and Daniel B. Carr

Jane is a 92-year-old female who presented to the emergency department with severe nociceptive pain subsequently diagnosed as an acute vertebral compression fracture. Her postoperative pain was well-controlled with an opioid-containing regimen, however, upon discharge, her orthopedic surgeon declined to give her a prescription for an opioid analgesic for use at home, citing concern that she would become addicted to the medication. Notably, however, Jane has no specific risk factors for opioid use disorder. Specifically, she has never smoked tobacco, nor does she drink alcohol or have a history of misusing other medications, cannabis, or illicit drugs. None of her family members misused opioids or other substances. Jane's chronic pharmacotherapy is limited to a multivitamin and 50 mcg levothyroxine, each taken daily. She does not use benzodiazepines nor does she take opioids chronically. Furthermore, none of her family members developed a substance use disorder. Last, Jane was not sexually abused as a preadolescent child, and she has no history of attention-deficit, obsessive-compulsive, or bipolar disorders, schizophrenia, or major depression.

What do you do now?

INTRODUCTION

Pain is a common reason for individuals to seek medical care, accounting for more than 6 million office visits in 2018 and more than 16 million emergency department visits in 2019.[1,2] During the past several decades, there have been numerous reports of undertreated pain in a wide variety of populations. Pain contributes to a broad spectrum of adverse outcomes, including unnecessary suffering, increased medical resource use, and impaired healing. Suboptimally managed acute pain is a risk factor for developing chronic pain. To complicate matters further, opioids—mainly illicit fentanyl—are currently associated with a staggering number of deaths in the United States each year.

DRUG SELECTION AND CLINICAL PRACTICE GUIDELINES

Medications are the cornerstone of pain management, and opioids are a component of this foundation. The choice of whether to prescribe an opioid, as well as the specific drug and dose chosen, depends on a careful risk–benefit analysis incorporating factors including the patient's clinical characteristics, the goals of therapy, and the prescriber's choices. The World Health Organization (WHO) analgesic ladder is a useful guide to help clinicians choose between medications across classes (Figure 19.1).[3]

The safe and effective use of opioids for different types of pain has been addressed in numerous guidelines[4-6] for postoperative, cancer-related, and chronic non-cancer pain. The 2022 National Comprehensive Cancer Network *Adult Cancer Pain* clinical practice guideline[7] highlights that improved survival is associated with effective pain and symptom management and that pain management is an essential part of cancer management. This guideline also provides recommendations for pain management in individuals with coexisting substance use disorders. In addition, opioid analgesics are included in the current WHO Model List of Essential Medicines.[8]

Despite their potential utility, even the most well-intended guidelines can be associated with unintended and potentially harmful consequences. In 2016, for instance, the Centers for Disease Control and Prevention (CDC) published a guideline for prescribing opioids for chronic pain.[9]

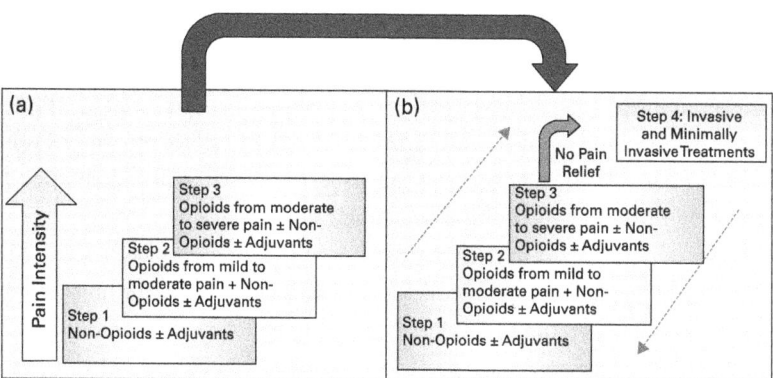

FIGURE 19.1 Transition from the original WHO three-step analgesic ladder (A) to the revised WHO fourth-step form (B). The additional step 4 is an "interventional" step and includes invasive and minimally invasive techniques. This updated WHO ladder provides a bidirectional approach.

Source: Reprinted from Cassella M. The revised WHO analgesic ladder © 2023, StatPearls Publishing LLC, Creative Commons CC-BY-NC-ND 4.0.

Recommendations contained in this publication—particularly those related to dose limits[10]—were widely adopted by clinicians, health systems, pharmacies, and insurers. This guideline was explicitly not intended for use in people with cancer, at the end of life, with painful conditions such as sickle cell disease, or individuals on methadone or buprenorphine maintenance. Their inappropriate application, including forced involuntary tapering, occurred with resulting patient harm, including deaths.[11–20] This guideline was updated in 2022.[11,12] It remains to be seen whether the new version will replace the older version in clinical practice, or how insurers and regulators will update their reimbursement and dispensing policies.

RISK OF OPIOID USE DISORDER

The likelihood that a person will develop a substance use disorder is a complex function of genetics, environment, and use of a reinforcing substance.[21] A key issue is how to apply population-level estimates of risk to individuals in order to provide safe and effective analgesia.

In their 2003 review, Ballantyne and Mao[22] made several important observations: (1) The biomedical literature on opioid therapy is largely based on lower quality evidence, such as surveys and uncontrolled and/or retrospective case series; (2) "patients with chronic pain not associated with a terminal disease can achieve satisfactory analgesia by using a stable (non-escalating) dose of opioids, with a minimal risk of addiction" (p. 1944); and (3) tolerance to analgesia may be associated with environmental and psychological factors in addition to biologic adaptation.

More recent data support these observations.[23] For example, in the 2016 CDC guideline on prescribing opioids for chronic pain,[9] the authors noted that in contrast to estimates suggesting high rates of prevalence of opioid use disorder in persons using prescribed opioids, rates of opioid abuse or dependence diagnosis (using *International Classification of Diseases, Ninth Revision, Clinical Modification* codes) ranged from 0.7% with lower dose (≤36 daily morphine milligram equivalents [MME]) chronic therapy to 6.1% with higher dose (≥120 MME) chronic therapy, versus 0.004% with no opioids prescribed. In primary care settings, the prevalence of opioid dependence (using the fourth edition of the *Diagnostic and Statistical Manual of Mental Disorders*) criteria ranged from 3% to 26%, whereas the prevalence of addiction in pain clinic patients ranged from 2% to 14%. In a 2018 report, the National Institute on Drug Abuse noted that although prescription opioid use and abuse are risk factors for heroin use, heroin use was rare.[24] Specifically, using data from 2002–2012—a period that corresponds to the escalation of the public health emergency associated with prescription opioids—0.39% of study respondents who reported previous nonmedical analgesic use began using heroin, compared to 0.02% of respondents who did not report prior nonmedical use. The wide range of these and related attempts at estimates speaks to the heterogeneous nature of this literature and of complexity involved with understanding the relation between opioid use and opioid use disorder.

EFFECTIVENESS OF OPIOID THERAPY FOR CHRONIC PAIN

There is also some uncertainty about the degree to which opioids are useful for chronic non-cancer pain. Two recent reports illustrate the state of our current understanding, as well as the difficulties inherent in understanding the estimates. In 2020, Chou et al.[25] assessed the effectiveness and harms of long-term opioid therapy, alternative opioid dosing strategies, and risk mitigation strategies. They found that opioids are associated with small improvements in pain and function versus placebo and increased risk of harm in the first 6 months of treatment. Evidence relating to long-term effectiveness is very limited, and the risk of harms may be dose-dependent, as noted in the 2016 CDC guideline.[9] In the short term, there were no differences between opioids and non-opioid medications in pain, function, mental health status, sleep, or depression. Coprescription of benzodiazepines and gabapentinoids may increase the risk of overdose. Overall, however, there was insufficient evidence to conclude whether opioids were effective for reducing pain and improving functioning over the long term.

In 2021, Nadeau et al.[26] reviewed this literature and noted evidence of opioid efficacy in terms of improved pain relief and physical functioning, as well as significant opioid-related side effects observed in randomized, placebo-controlled trials. In general, however, these trials do not account for interpatient variability in opioid dose or address titration to adequate control of pain. Furthermore, estimates of the risk of death from opioid treatment are limited by not accounting for the source of prescribed opioids (e.g., in a legitimate therapeutic clinical relationship vs. in medically unsupervised use, such as from "pill mills"). Last, a large proportion of people who report using heroin at least once also report using opioids nonmedically at least once. As a result, generalizing from studies of people with complex histories of drug use to the population at large can contribute to an inaccurate conclusion that any prescription of opioids, no matter how short, is associated with a high risk of developing an opioid use disorder.

RISK FACTORS FOR MISUSE AND SERIOUS ADVERSE EVENTS

Consensus recommendations in the 2022 CDC guideline[11,12] include the following salient points: (1) Factors that may vary over time (e.g., alcohol use and concomitant pharmacotherapy) should be evaluated frequently; and (2) sleep-disordered breathing, a history of overdose or substance use disorder, use of at least 50 MME per day, and concurrent use of benzodiazepines are considered important risk factors for harm. Individuals with these characteristics should be assessed frequently, naloxone should be offered to them and their social contacts, and they should be instructed in its use. In addition, pregnancy, renal or hepatic insufficiency, age 65 years or older, working in safety critical occupations, and suboptimal treatment of mental health conditions should be considered as part of the decision regarding whether to prescribe opioids for chronic pain.

CASE RESOLUTION

How should we apply the previously discussed recommendations to the patient in our case? She presents with new onset of acute pain secondary to an acute vertebral compression fracture—pain that may be reasonably expected to respond to opioids. Her risk factors are limited to advanced age and possibly some age-related diminution of renal function, yet these characteristics do not suggest an increased risk of addiction. She has no history of conditions that are potential risk factors for a substance use disorder. Despite this, the orthopedic surgeon remains hesitant to prescribe an opioid analgesic because of a perceived risk of addiction. Despite a low risk of opioid-related harm, caution is still warranted. However, the goal is to provide optimal analgesia safely and effectively during the self-limited time before the vertebral compression fracture stabilizes and the associated pain subsides. The goal is not to categorically refuse to use to the tools we have at our disposal when they are indicated clinically. Baseline and follow-up assessments of risk are important. As noted in the 2022 CDC guideline,[11,12] reassessments should be more frequent for factors that are potentially time-varying, including use of concurrent medications, new diagnoses, changes in physical and emotional status, and use of substances such as nicotine and alcohol.

The clinician should be careful to prescribe medication at a pharmacokinetically appropriate dose and schedule. The concept of "start low, go slow" is applicable here. Most regular-release opioids provide analgesia for approximately 3 hours, on average. Yet, dosing intervals of 4–6 hours or even longer are commonly used, forcing the patient with consistent pain to wait and watch the clock until the next dose is scheduled. Morphine has an active metabolite (morphine-6-glucuronide) that is eliminated renally, so it should be used cautiously in persons with diminished renal function. In addition, codeine and tramadol must be metabolized to their active metabolites (morphine and O-desmethyl-tramadol, respectively) by cytochrome P450 2D6, which is subject to genetic polymorphism. Rapid metabolizers are expected to generate higher levels of these metabolites and are at increased risk for adverse events (although not necessarily increased risk of addiction), whereas slow metabolizers may not generate enough active metabolite to provide analgesia. Tramadol can be challenging to use because it interferes with serotonin and norepinephrine reuptake, making this drug a little like using an opioid and an antidepressant at the same time. Finally, long-acting opioids are contraindicated in opioid-naive individuals.

KEY POINTS TO REMEMBER

· Opioid analgesics are important components of the analgesic toolkit. However, their safe and effective use in medically supervised settings during the public health crisis of illicit and illegal opioid use (particularly fentanyl) is often complicated by stigma related to an exaggerated fear of addiction in such settings.

· Assessment and understanding the multifactorial nature of opioid use disorder and opioids' pharmacological and pharmacokinetic characteristics can help prescribers and patients achieve optimal analgesia while reducing risk.

References

1. National Center for Health Statistics. National Ambulatory Medical Care Survey: 2018 national summary tables. 2018. https://www.cdc.gov/nchs/data/ahcd/namcs_summary/2018-namcs-web-tables-508.pdf

2. National Center for Health Statistics. National Hospital Ambulatory Medical Care Survey: 2019 emergency department summary tables. 2019. https://www.cdc.gov/nchs/data/nhamcs/web_tables/2019-nhamcs-ed-web-tables-508.pdf

3. Anekar AA, Cascella M. WHO analgesic ladder. In *StatPearls*. StatPearls. Updated May 15, 2022. https://www.ncbi.nlm.nih.gov/books/NBK554435

4. Chou R, Gordon DB, de Leon-Casasola OA, et al. Management of postoperative pain: A clinical practice guideline from the American Pain Society, the American Society of Regional Anesthesia and Pain Medicine, and the American Society of Anesthesiologists' Committee on Regional Anesthesia, Executive Committee, and Administrative Council. *J Pain*. 2016;17(2):131–157. https://doi.org/10.1016/j.jpain.2015.12.008

5. Coccolini F, Corradi F, Sartelli M, et al. Postoperative pain management in non-traumatic emergency general surgery: WSES–GAIS–SIAARTI–AAST guidelines. *World J Emerg Surg.* 2022;17(1):50. doi:10.1186/s13017-022-00455-7

6. Strassels SA, McNicol E, Suleman R. Postoperative pain management: A practical review, Part 1. *Am J Health Syst Pharm.* 2005;62(18):1904–1916. doi:10.2146/ajhp040490.p1

7. National Comprehensive Cancer Network. Adult cancer pain (Version 2.2022). 2022. Accessed September 24, 2022. https://www.nccn.org/professionals/physic ian_gls/pdf/pain.pdf

8. World Health Organization. WHO Model Lists of Essential Medicines. 2022. Accessed September 28, 2022. https://www.who.int/groups/expert-committee-on-selection-and-use-of-essential-medicines/essential-medicines-lists

9. Dowell D, Haegerich TM, Chou R. CDC guideline for prescribing opioids for chronic pain—United States, 2016. *MMWR Recomm Rep.* 2016;65(1):1-49. doi:10.15585/mmwr.rr6501e1

10. Dowell D, Compton WM, Giroir BP. Patient-centered reduction or discontinuation of long-term opioid analgesics: The HHS guide for clinicians. *JAMA.* 2019;322(19):1855–1856. doi:10.1001/jama.2019.16409

11. Dowell D, Ragan KR, Jones CM, Baldwin GT, Chou R. CDC clinical practice guideline for prescribing opioids for pain—United States, 2022. *MMWR Recomm Rep.* 2022;71(3):1–95. doi:10.15585/mmwr.rr7103a1

12. Dowell D, Ragan KR, Jones CM, Baldwin GT, Chou R. Prescribing opioids for pain: The new CDC clinical practice guideline. *N Engl J Med.* 2022;387(22):2011–2013. doi:10.1056/NEJMp2211040

13. Dowell D, Haegerich T, Chou R. No shortcuts to safer opioid prescribing. *N Engl J Med.* 2019;380(24):2285–2287. doi:10.1056/NEJMp1904190

14. Dowell D, Noonan RK, Houry D. Underlying factors in drug overdose deaths. *JAMA.* 2017;318(23):2295–2296. doi:10.1001/jama.2017.15971

15. Kroenke K, Alford DP, Argoff C, et al. Challenges with implementing the Centers for Disease Control and Prevention opioid guideline: A consensus panel report. *Pain Med.* 2019;20(4):724–735. doi:10.1093/pm/pny307

16. U.S. Food and Drug Administration. FDA identifies harm reported from sudden discontinuation of opioid pain medicines and requires label changes to guide prescribers on gradual, individualized tapering. US Department of Health and Human Services, Food and Drug Administration. 2019. Accessed March 16, 2023. https://www.fda.gov/drugs/drug-safety-and-availability/fda-identifies-harm-repor ted-sudden-discontinuation-opioid-pain-medicines-and-requires-label-changes

17. Demidenko MI, Dobscha SK, Morasco BJ, Meath THA, Ilgen MA, Lovejoy TI. Suicidal ideation and suicidal self-directed violence following clinician-initiated prescription opioid discontinuation among long-term opioid users. *Gen Hosp Psychiatry.* 2017;47:29–35. doi:10.1016/j.genhosppsych.2017.04.011

18. Coffin PO, Rowe C, Oman N, et al. Illicit opioid use following changes in opioids prescribed for chronic non-cancer pain. *PLoS One.* 2020;15(5):e0232538. doi:10.1371/journal.pone.0232538

19. Rowe CL, Eagen K, Ahern J, Faul M, Hubbard A, Coffin P. Evaluating the effects of opioid prescribing policies on patient outcomes in a safety-net primary care clinic. *J Gen Intern Med.* 2022;37(1):117–124. doi:10.1007/s11606-021-06920-4

20. Mark TL, Parish W. Opioid medication discontinuation and risk of adverse opioid-related health care events. *J Subst Abuse Treat.* 2019;103:58–63. doi:10.1016/j.jsat.2019.05.001

21. Savage SR, Joranson DE, Covington EC, Schnoll SH, Heit HA, Gilson AM. Definitions related to the medical use of opioids: Evolution towards universal agreement. *J Pain Symptom Manage.* 2003;26(1):655–667. doi:10.1016/s0885-3924(03)00219-7

22. Ballantyne JC, Mao J. Opioid therapy for chronic pain. *N Engl J Med.* 2003;349(20):1943–1953. doi:10.1056/NEJMra025411

23. Keyes KM, Rutherford C. Prevalence of addiction in chronic pain: Reanalysis of Vowles et al., 2015. *Pain.* 2022;163(5):e693–e695. doi:10.1097/j.pain.0000000000002573

24. National Institute on Drug Abuse. Prescription opioids and heroin report. 2018. Accessed October 12, 2022. https://nida.nih.gov/publications/research-reports/prescription-opioids-heroin

25. Chou R, Hartung D, Turner J, et al. *Opioid treatments for chronic pain.* Comparative Effectiveness Review No. 229. Agency for Healthcare Research and Quality. 2020. https://www.ncbi.nlm.nih.gov/books/NBK556253/pdf/Bookshelf_NBK556253.pdf

26. Nadeau SE, Wu JK, Lawhern RA. Opioids and chronic pain: An analytic review of the clinical evidence. *Front Pain Res.* 2021;2:721357. doi:10.3389/fpain.2021.721357

20 The Emerging Role of Independent Patient Advocates

Shiella Dowlatshahi

A 30 year-old clinician with a history of melanoma at age 20, then resolved by surgery, was discharged after emergency excisional biopsy of a recurrent suspicious thigh lesion. Culture identified a "flesh-eating" bacterial infection. A suction wound drain was placed predischarge and continued along with outpatient intravenous antibiotics for six weeks, then discontinued as local healing was well under way. Ongoing moderate-to-severe pain at the incision, and an antalgic gait, were present at hospital discharge and persisted. When reaching out to arrange follow up with her primary care provider, she learned that person had left their practice and their replacement was fully booked for at least four months.

Pre-discharge consensus was that she would benefit from further ongoing evaluation by a neurologist, rehabilitation specialist, and pain specialist. Although the patient worked in the same institution where she received care, she found appointments hard to schedule in a timely fashion. Her insuror sent her multiple confusing forms. Not knowing what to do or whom to turn to, she was intrigued to hear from a relative about a recently evolving support role ("independent patient advocate"). She reached out to such a practitioner.

What do you do now?

DISCUSSION

The case involves a 30-year-old individual seeking care after being discharged from the hospital. Alarmingly, although this patient was a health care professional herself, she found it difficult to access appropriate care for several issues that were unresolved. Unfortunately, this is all too common in the current dysfunctional health care system, where continuity of care is disrupted due to a lack of follow-up, provider inertia, bewildering complexity, and limited access to care in a shrinking industry. Challenges to the U.S. health care system are well recognized. Despite progress in health care delivery and advancements in treatments, neither patients nor providers are satisfied with the current state of health care, which is inefficient, expensive, and confers no comparative benefits over other countries' outcomes.[1] Efforts have been made to address existing issues. Yet these efforts have largely failed. Some of these measures include the introduction of value-based care, patient navigators, and artificial intelligence integration.[2] These measures often dilute or remove the human element, increase the use of profit-centered metrics over patient-centered care, and increase provider burden and frustration, leading to burnout. To add to the complexities, patients often receive voluminous paperwork and bills from different providers with varying contractual relationships with insurance companies, leaving them feeling dissatisfied with their medical care and frustrated and confused with the paperwork they need to sift through to reconcile billing statements. In this case, the patient decided to enlist independent third-party assistance to help guide her through the post-discharge period and cumbersome insurance paperwork.

It is concerning that in the current health care system in the United States, even health care professionals may encounter challenges in obtaining timely access to care. The profession of independent patient advocate is expanding, driven by growing demand for professionals who act on behalf of patients to resolve complex issues relating to patient care. As health care needs grow in the United States, and shortages of physicians and other providers continue, it will be even more important for patients to advocate for themselves through a third-party professional. Independent patient advocates do not subscribe to a single institution only, nor are they tied into a health care system. A proficient and knowledgeable independent patient advocate can actively champion the patient's needs by eliminating access barriers, facilitating seamless communication among health care providers, ensuring smooth transitions across health care settings, and providing invaluable assistance with insurance paperwork and billing. Most important, the approach of an independent patient advocate is fundamentally patient-centric, characterized by respect for the patient's preferences and commitment to prioritizing the patient's individual needs.

THE ROLE OF AN INDEPENDENT PATIENT ADVOCATE

Like the patient in this case, patients are often discharged without adequate post-hospitalization care plans or clear instructions, creating a gap in care that may contribute to worsening conditions, readmissions, or additional health complications, consequently escalating health care expenses. Miscommunication or incomplete information during the transition process may also result in medication errors, such as incorrect dosages or missed prescriptions. In addition, if discharge instructions are incomplete, patients may struggle with managing their conditions or may miss vital information about necessary follow-up care. This case highlights inadequate planning and a lack of coordination among health care providers, resulting in the patient lacking essential ongoing support required to optimally manage their health.

In this scenario, an independent patient advocate can play a pivotal role in fostering communication with the surgeon's office and identifying suitable rehabilitation, neurology, and pain management specialists. The advocate will ideally communicate with primary care providers or concierge medicine practices in the area to coordinate a follow-up visit and develop a comprehensive care plan. The patient advocate can additionally liaise with the primary care office to facilitate the seamless transfer of the patient's records to their new primary care or concierge physician. In case of outstanding insurance bills, an independent patient advocate can play a pivotal role in addressing billing concerns, negotiating discrepancies or overcharges, and frequently achieving reductions in patients' medical bills.

The role of an independent patient advocate is continuously evolving in response to growing demand for individuals who can adeptly navigate the intricate landscape of the current health care system on behalf of patients.

CHOOSING AN INDEPENDENT PATIENT ADVOCATE

To find the right independent patient advocate, patients should consider several factors. It is essential to look for advocates with relevant experience and expertise in the specific area of concern. Advocates can have varying backgrounds, including health care law, health care practice, nursing, social work, and so on. In addition, Board Certification in Patient Advocacy (BCPA) can also be an indication of a qualified advocate. More than half of the respondents to a patient survey expressed they would prefer to work with an advocate with board certification.[3] This credentialing is also important to health care providers, who feel more positively about working with credentialed patient support personnel.

The BCPA credential program began in 2018. It allows patient advocates to assess their knowledge and skills and to show their understanding of the ethical standards involved in advocacy.[4] Currently, several academic institutions offer a curriculum in patient advocacy. Patient advocacy organizations, such as the Alliance of Professional Health Advocates, Umbra Health, and Greater National Advocates can serve as valuable resources for patients seeking assistance with clinical decisions, follow-up, insurance, and billing issues.[3]

Choosing an independent patient advocate utilizing one of the organizations mentioned above may be a useful first step. Through these organizations, one can identify an advocate with relevant experience. References from previous patients and their experience may also be helpful in choosing an advocate. Although not necessary, certifications are helpful when identifying advocates. An initial consultation with a potential advocate should be scheduled to discuss specific needs; the approach; experience; pricing; availability; and the "chemistry" between patient, family, and advocate. Most independent patient advocates will have an hourly rate or retainer paid directly by the patient. A small percentage of advocates offer package pricing. Nearly 25% of advocates in one study reported doing pro bono practices.[3]

Once the patient advocate is selected, it is important to establish clear goals, timelines, expectations, and scope of services in a written document or contract to avoid misunderstanding regarding the expected outcomes. Patients and their families should collaborate with the patient advocate by providing any pertinent medical records, test results, or relevant documentation related to their case. This step is essential for the advocate to gain a comprehensive understanding of the situation and advocate effectively on the patient's behalf. Together, patients and families should actively engage with the patient advocate to develop a well-defined action plan. Advocates can act as intermediaries, enhancing communication between patients, their families, and health care professionals, as well as gathering additional information and ensuring that any concerns are promptly addressed. Maintaining regular and open communication with the patient advocate is of utmost importance to regularly assess progress and address any emerging challenges that may arise.

CASE RESOLUTION

In the case presented in this chapter, the patient and her family retained an independent patient advocate when confronted with seemingly insurmountable administrative issues, including scheduling and bundling timely outpatient appointments post-discharge. Doing so permitted more prompt and efficient attention to her medical needs, including wound care and rehabilitation. The patient and her family were satisfied their involvement of an independent patient advocate accelerated her return to normal function. Independent patient advocates offer indispensable support by providing personalized patient-centered care to ensure optimal health care experiences. An independent patient advocate can play a crucial role in preserving the health and safety of patients and improving outcomes while reducing hospitalizations. This is particularly important for individuals from lower socioeconomic classes who may face barriers to follow-up care and struggle with the burdensome costs of health care. By providing support, coordination, and advocacy, patient advocates can help bridge these gaps and ensure that patients receive the care they need, ultimately leading to better health outcomes.

KEY POINTS TO REMEMBER

· The current model of health care has made it increasingly necessary but also more difficult for physicians and allied health professionals to advocate for their patients.

- Collaboration with an independent patient advocate is an important option to help ensure timely, patient-centered care.
- Although the services of a dedicated independent patient advocate may not serve as a panacea to remedy all issues within the health care system, this still-emerging role reintroduces the crucial human element into a system that often lacks it.

References

1. Abel B, et al. Patient satisfaction: A critical indicator of healthcare quality. Open Access. 2017.
2. Dowlatshahi S. *Pack Your Own Healthcare Parachute: A Physician's Death Through His Daughter's Eyes.* 10-10-10 Publishing; 2022.
3. Coalition of Health Care Advocacy Organizations. [Home page].2023. https://chcao.org
4. Christo L, Droppert B, Kempton C, et al. The critical role of patient and health care advocates: A special report. Coalition of Health Care Advocacy Organizations. 2023. https://chcao.org/special-report-2023

Further Reading

Dean W, Talbot S, Dean A. Reframing clinician distress: Moral injury not burnout. *Fed Pract Health Care.* 2019;36(9):400–402.

Ducharme J. Long waits, short appointments, huge bills: U.S. health care is causing patient burnout. *Time.* February 27, 2023.

Farber NJ. Why you need a patient advocate in the hospital. *U.S. News & World Report,* June 8, 2017.

Kurani N, Wager E. How does the quality of the U.S. health system compare to other countries? Peterson-KFF Health System Tracker; 2023.

Saad L. Americans sour on the U.S. healthcare quality. Gallup.com; January 19, 2023.

Shmerling RH. Is our healthcare system broken? Harvard Health; July 13, 2021.

21 Managing Outpatient Workplace Violence

Pragya B. Gupta and Daniel B. Carr

Mrs. Brown was admitted with fever and leukopenia 3 months following stem cell transplant. Despite appropriate therapy, her sepsis is progressing. Due to their anger at what they perceive is insufficient responsiveness to her needs leading to a bad outcome, the patient's son and nephew are making threats to the physical well-being of the staff.

What do you do now?

INTRODUCTION

Hammurabi's code (circa 1800 BCE) instructed society to reward or punish healers based on their outcomes. By 400 BCE, Hippocratic-era authors recognized that physicians are often blamed quickly, even when poor outcomes are expected.[1] Currently, these themes play out amid a backdrop of high expectations for excellent outcomes by patients, families, and the public and easy access to lethal weapons in many countries. Accordingly, physicians, nurses, social workers, physical therapists, pharmacists, and other health care workers (HCWs) are increasingly subject to fatal and nonfatal injuries.

DEFINITION AND CLASSIFICATION

The National Institute of Occupational Safety and Health (NIOSH) defines workplace violence (WPV) as any physical assault, threatening behavior, or verbal abuse occurring in the workplace.[2] NIOSH classifies workplace violence into four types, as shown in Table 21.1.

WPV PREVALENCE AND INTERVENTION TRIALS

Current literature on WPV emphasizes those in the outpatient health care setting because inpatients are more frail and less mobile than outpatients. Multiple authors have commented on the paucity of high-quality research on WPV in health care clinics, making detailed analysis and consolidation of their contents unfeasible.[3-6] However, descriptive statistics paint a picture of an already huge and still growing problem.

HCWs accounted for 73% of the 1.3 million nonfatal workplace injuries and illnesses due to violence in 2018.[7,8] The average annual victimization rate from nonfatal WPV during 2015–2019 for physicians was 15.1 per 1,000, followed by 26.3 per 1,000 for nurses and 46.1 per 1,000 for social workers/psychiatrists.[8] Because the U.S. Bureau of Labor Statistics does not record verbal incidents, the prevalence of WPV cannot be reliably gauged based on data from this agency.[5] Some have recommended that verbal abuse be recognized as WPV because verbal assault is a risk factor for battery.[5] Odes et al.[6] collected data from the California Occupational Safety and Health Administration (Cal/OSHA) through the WPV incidents

TABLE 21.1 **Workplace Violence**

Type	Description	Examples
1	Criminal intent: No relationship with the business or its employee.	Less common in a health care setting. It is usually committing a crime in conjunction with robbery, trespassing, shoplifting, etc.
2	Client on worker violence: Clients include patients, family members, and visitors.	Most common type. Frequently seen in the emergency department, psychiatry units, waiting rooms, and geriatric settings. Verbal abuse is most common.
3	Lateral or horizontal Violence: Includes bullying, vindictive actions, humiliating, and unfair verbal and emotional abuse up to homicide.	Supervisor to supervisee, physician to nurse, or peer to peer.
4	Violence centering on personal relationship: The perpetrator has a personal relationship with the nurse outside work that spills over to the work environment.	The husband of a nurse follows her to work, orders her home, and threatens her, with implications for not only this nurse but also for her co-workers and patients.

Adapted from Centers for Disease Control and Prevention (https://wwwn.cdc.gov/WPVHC/Nurses/Course/Slide/Unit1_5).

reporting system from July 1, 2017, through September 30, 2018. They found patients to be aggressors 93% of the time, and 75% of emergency department (ED) nurses and 85% of psychiatry nurses experienced WPV monthly or more frequently.

Groenewold et al.[9] analyzed WPV injury surveillance data submitted by 106 hospitals participating in the Occupational Health Safety Network, a Web-based system created by NIOSH for hospitals, from 2012 to 2015 and found that data were frequently missing for important variables. The study found that most WPVs in hospitals are type 2. Nurses and nursing assistants (40.2%) sustained the most WPV. Females suffered the majority of injuries (66.4%). A total of 48.3% of all injuries resulted in lost workdays. Patients were the perpetrators in 94.8% of cases. Of all WPVs, 98.5% were physical assaults. A total of 60% of WPVs occurred where direct patient care was performed, including the patient's room.[9] Clinicians practicing pain medicine frequently experience actual or threatened WPV.[3] Threats and violence commonly surround opioid management and worker's compensation. Patient factors leading to violence were intoxication, decompensated mental health (e.g., depression and psychosocial distress), and dissatisfaction with care. Clinics with poor violence control programs had a higher rate of verbal threats.[3]

The only systematic review that examined WPV in health clinics found that the prevalence of type 2 WPV ranged from 9% to 74.5%.[4] Verbal abuse was the most common at 42.1–94.3%. The threat of assault was 14–57%, bullying 2.5–5.7%, physical assault 0.5–15.9%, intimidation 22%, and sexual assault and harassment 0.2–9.3%. Of the physicians, 24.4–59.3% reported experiencing WPV, nurses reported a frequency of 9.5–62.1%, receptionists reported 15.1–68.4%, and technicians reported 24.5–40%. The study also found that rural clinics had higher WPV rates than urban locations. Evening or night shifts (64.1%) had more WPV than morning shifts (38%). The perpetrators were usually patients (71.5%) rather than companions (28.1%).[4]

Shiozaki et al.[10] administered questionnaires nationwide to 1,225 bereaved family members of patients with cancer who died in a palliative care unit in Japan. The main reasons for family dissatisfaction were a lack of perceived support for maintaining hope, lack of perceived respect for individuality, perception of poor quality of care, inadequate staffing, unavailability of timely admission to the palliative care unit, lack of accurate information about palliative care units, and family financial burden.[10]

Hinchey et al.[11] conducted a prospective cohort study of patients in a primary care clinic. They explored patient–physician characteristics associated with being considered "difficult" and assessed the impact on patient outcomes. Among 750 subjects, 133 (17.8%) were perceived as difficult. The study found that difficult patients were less likely to trust the physician; not fully satisfied with their clinician; and more likely to have worsening symptoms at 2 weeks, more than five symptoms, a history of recent stress, and depression or anxiety disorder. Physicians involved in difficult encounters were less experienced with psychosocial orientation scores on the Physician Belief Scale (PBS), a measure of willingness to deal with the psychosocial aspects of medicine. Clinicians with a low score on the PBS have a more open communication style and lower liability claims rates.[11]

WPV in health care is linked to HCW burnout. ED personnel are at high risk for WPV. Vrablik et al.[12] conducted a prospective qualitative study with semistructured interviews of 23 HCWs within 24 hours of WPV events: 39% of participants were nurses, and 9% were physicians. No physical abuse was reported. Based on their observations, Vrablik et al. recommended using cognitive–behavioral techniques for the emergency room staff before their shift to strengthen their coping mechanisms and thereby reduce burnout rates.[12] Burnout is associated with more medical errors, suboptimal patient care, diminished emotional and physical well-being, diminished sense of personal and professional accomplishment, increased absenteeism, and job turnover.

Gillespie et al.[13] studied the implementation of a multidisciplinary intervention to reduce physical assault and threats in the ED. The study included two EDs of a level 1 trauma center, two urban tertiary care EDs, and two community-based suburban EDs. A total of 209 participants were used for statistical analysis. Three survey tools were used: demographic survey, the number of assaults and threats during the previous months collated through email, and The Violent Event Survey (details of assailant and the event using the Violent Event Survey). The intervention involved three EDs exposed to three components: environmental changes, policies and procedures, and education and training. Control EDs did not implement these interventions. Although the intervention reduced the incidence of WPV, there were no significant differences in assault or physical threat rates according to gender, occupation, and ED type.[13]

A well-designed randomized controlled trial by Arnetz et al.[14] evaluated the impact of the data-driven intervention in reducing type 2 WPV by prospectively tracking the population-based incidence rate of patient-to-worker violence and related injury. The study mandated that all type 2 WPV be entered into the hospital's electronic reporting system, which was de-identified and used to calculate the incidence rate of WPV per 100 full-time equivalent. The project required active collaboration with hospital system representatives of occupational health, safety, nursing, security, human resources, and labor. The study comprised four phases:

Phase 1: Development of a standardized report of WPV with information on rates of violence, injuries, and description of violence based on incident reports.

Phase 2: Implementing the Hazard Matrix[15] to prioritize hospital units for interventions. The matrix identified hospital work units at increased risk for violence.

Phase 3: Randomized interventions. Pairs of units were randomized to intervention or control. The intervention was a "walk through" or worksite visit. During the visit, the units were apprised of their WPV data compared to the overall hospital data.

Phase 4: Intervention outcome evaluation—across 5 years. Data were collected pre- and post-intervention at 6-month intervals.

At 24 months, the incidence rate ratio for the intervention group decreased from 2.33 (confidence interval [CI]: 1.41, 3.84) to 0.37 (CI: 0.46, 1.63), whereas in the non-intervention group, WPV increased from 2.81 to 3.43. The overall result suggests a positive effect of the intervention in reducing violent events and their severity, whereas in the control group, violence increased. Despite the overall increase in violence rate in the U.S. population by the end of the 5-year period, there were no statistically significant changes in injury rates. The decrease in type 2 violent injury in this study population was attributed to the data-driven interventions (e.g., educating staff to de-escalate violent events). This study highlighted applying the interventions at the unit level, which motivated the supervisors of the units to assume ownership. This study was flexible, allowing each unit to have its own prevention strategies. However, the outcome did not achieve statistical significance.[14]

Team Strategies and Tools to Enhance Performance and Patient Safety (TeamSTEPPS),[16] developed by the Agency for Healthcare Research and Department of Defense, was released in 2006 as a national standard for team training in health care. It introduces tools and strategies to improve team performance in health care. The training underscores the reduction of WPV through early intervention and enhances staff and patient experience and satisfaction by building a culture of patient safety and staff safety. The program educates employees on the early detection of WPV symptoms, de-escalation techniques, reporting of WPV, and proper documentation of incidents. It trains employees to identify nonverbal signs of impending violence, such as rapid eye movements, pacing, rapid breathing, altered facial expression, gestures, and postures such as clenching of jaws and fists.[16]

RISK FACTORS FOR WPV

Patient-Related Factors

Multiple studies have found that in 90% of cases, patients tend to be aggressors, and in only 10–20% of cases are visitors and/or relatives the perpetrators of violence. Patient-related factors are dissatisfaction with care, poorly controlled pain, substance use disorder, psychiatric illnesses such as depression, personality disorder, intoxication, altered mental status associated with dementia, delirium, delusion, and decompensated mental state. In chronic pain care settings, factors include opioid management issues, workers' compensation-related issues, litigation, and patients being forced to see third-party physicians (particularly worker's compensation patients). Other factors are failure to receive work or sick notes from clinicians, sexual abuse, poverty, the presence of weapons, and gang activity. Patients in police custody are at risk for WPV (one study reported a 29% incidence of shooting in the emergency room and 11% violence during escape),[5] communication problems with caregivers (language barrier or illiteracy), and difficulty comprehending and accepting bad news related to diagnosis and prognosis.

Clinic Setting–Related Risk Factors

Clinic setting–related risk factors include unmet service needs, medical/clerical errors, overcrowding, long wait times, uncomfortable lounges, understaffing, and high staff turnover. Working alone in a facility can place clinicians at risk for WPV. Poor environmental design impedes escape from violent crime. Location of a clinic in neighborhoods with a high crime rate poses a risk for WPV; however, rural clinics have higher WPV rates than urban clinics. Unrestricted movement of the public in clinics and hospitals and inadequate or absent security personnel also predispose HCWs to WPV.

CONSEQUENCES OF WPV

Consequences of WPV include HCW burnout, anxiety, fear, helplessness, reduced job satisfaction, depression, chronic fatigue, anger, feeling unsafe, physical injury, actual stress reaction, post-traumatic stress disorder, and the need for psychological support.[12] Consequences of burnout are increased medical error, suboptimal patient care, diminished emotional or physical well-being, diminished feelings of personal or professional accomplishment, increased absenteeism, and job turnover.

PREVENTION OF WPV

There are no evidence-based guidelines for preventing WPV. Many authors suggest there should be zero tolerance for verbal abuse and that it should be reported to the supervisor and security personnel/local law enforcement immediately.[4-6,14] Tolerance of low-level crime often leads to more serious crime.[5] All clinic staff should receive training in aggression de-escalation and self-defense techniques and recognize early nonverbal signs of anxiety, stress, and impending violence in patients or relatives.[13,14,16] Chart flagging has successfully prevented WPV in the Veterans Administration health care system. Implementing cognitive behavioral techniques for clinic staff before starting the clinic/shift can reduce WPV.[12] Implementation of interventions as suggested by Gillespie et al.[13] and Arnetz et al.,[14] as detailed above, may also reduce WPV. Rosenstein et al.[17] stressed that physicians should project a basic professional manner; see patients promptly; be direct, honest, and specific; and acknowledge limitations in clinicians' ability to predict treatment response and outcome.

Patients with substance/opioid use disorders should be evaluated using appropriate tools such as the Opioid Risk Tool, referred to an addiction specialist, and provided medication-assisted treatment per Substance Abuse and Mental Health Services Administration guidelines. Mental health support staff should always be available on-site.[5,13] Other measures include installing metal detectors, physical barriers such as a high countertop with an acrylic barrier, a duress alarm (sounds alarm and rings police), a paging system, and a lockdown system in the clinic. Implementation of the Cal/OSHA and Security Act has reduced the incidence of emergency room violence.[6]

CASE RESOLUTION

Based on the available literature and common sense, specific steps can be taken to preempt violence. The most experienced physicians in the office should deal with Mrs. Brown's family. Employment of an interdisciplinary team, rounding as a team, and prompt meetings with the family may de-escalate the situation. A consistent treatment plan should be promoted. Clinicians should be forthright with Mrs. Brown's family and set realistic expectations. The limitations of treatment should be explained empathetically. At the same time, physicians should be clear about the requirement for appropriate behavior by all in the clinic. The design of the clinic should incorporate physical safety measures, including barriers and silent alarms or panic buttons, for instances in which despite pre-emptive measures to avert WPV, it still occurs.

KEY POINTS TO REMEMBER

- WPV is pervasive and a significant public health issue.
- Verbal abuse should be reported promptly to the supervisor, security personnel, or local law enforcement.
- WPV is linked with HCW burnout, resulting in emotional distress, depression, job turnover, and diminished professional performance.
- Dissatisfaction with care is the key driver of WPV.
- Training in aggression de-escalation and self-defense techniques may reduce WPV.
- WPV is more likely in clinics located in high-crime areas.
- Less experienced physicians and physicians with low psychosocial orientation scores on the Patient Belief Scale tend to be involved in WPV more frequently.[11]

References

1. Papavramidou N, Vlulstos P. Medical malpractice cases in the Hippocratic collection: A review and today's perspective. *Hippokratia*. 2019;23(3):99–105.
2. National Institute for Occupational Safety and Health. Violence occupational hazards in hospitals. Publication no. 2002-101. U.S. Department of Health and Human Services, Centers for Disease Control and Prevention, National Institute

for Occupational Safety and Health. April 2002. https://www.cdc.gov/niosh/docs/2002-101/pdfs/2002-101.pdf?id=10.26616/NIOSHPUB2002101

3. Moman R, Maher PD, Hooten M. Workplace violence in the setting of pain management. *Mayo Clin Proc Innov Qual Outcomes.* 2020;4(2):211–215.

4. Pompeii L, Benavides E, Pop O, et al. Workplace violence in outpatient physician clinics: A systematic review. *Int J Environ Res Public Health.* 2020;17(18):6587.

5. Phillips J. Workplace violence against health care workers in the United States. *N Engl J Med.* 2016;374:1661–1669.

6. Odes R, Hong O, Harrison R, et al. Factors associated with physical injury or police involvement during incidents of workplace violence in hospitals: Findings from the first year of California's new standard. *Am J Ind Med.* 2020;63:543–549.

7. The Joint Commission. R3 report Issue 30: Workplace violence prevention standards. June 18, 2021. https://www.jointcommission.org/standards/r3-report/r3-report-issue-30-workplace-violence-prevention-standards

8. Harrell E, Langon L, Pegula SM, et al. Indicator of workplace violence 2019. NCJ 250748; NIOSH 2022-124. U.S. Department of Justice, Bureau of Justice Statistics; July 2022.

9. Groenewold MR, Sarmiento RFR, Vanoli K, Raudabaugh W, Nowlin S. Workplace violence injury in 106 US hospitals participating in the Occupational Health Safety Network (OHSN), 2012–2015. *Am J Ind Med.* 2018;61:157–166.

10. Shiozaki M, Morita T, Hirai K, Tsuneto S, Shima Y. Why are bereaved family members dissatisfied with specialized inpatient palliative care service? A nationwide qualitative study. *Palliat Med.* 2005;19:319–327.

11. Hinchey S, Jackson J. A cohort study assessing difficult patient encounters in a walk-in primary care clinic, predictors, and outcomes. *J Gen Intern Med.* 2011;26(6):588–594.

12. Vrablik CM, Chipman AK, Rosenman ED, et al. Identification of processes that mediate the impact of workplace violence on emergency department healthcare workers in the USA: Results from a qualitative study. *BMJ Open.* 2019;9e031781. doi:10.1136/bmjopen-2019-031781

13. Gillespie GL, Gates DM, Kowalenko T, Bresler S, Succop P. Implementation of a comprehensive intervention to reduce physical assaults and threats in the emergency department. *J Emerg Nurs.* 2014;40:586–591.

14. Arnetz JE, Hamblin L, Russell J, et al. Prevention of patient-to-worker violence in hospitals: Outcome of a randomized controlled intervention. *J Occup Environ Med.* 2017;59(1):18–27.

15. Centers for Disease Control and Prevention, National Institute for Occupation Safety and Health. Focus on prevention: Conducting a hazard risk assessment. 2003. http://www.cdc.gov/niosh.minig/userfiles/works/pdfs

16. Agency for Healthcare Research and Quality. TeamSTEPPS (Team Strategies & Tools to Enhance Performance & Patient Safety): Reducing workplace violence with TeamSTEPPS. https://www.ahrq.gov/teamstepps/index.html

17. Rosenstein DL, Block SD, Givens J. Challenging interaction with patients and families in palliative care. UpToDate. Updated May 23, 2024. https://www.uptod ate.com/contents/challenging-interactions-with-patients-and-families-in-palliat ive-care

22 MaladaptiveTeam Dynamics

Moe Norton-Westbrook, Sylvia Christie, and Constance Dahlin

Francisco Cruz is a 68-year-old Puerto Rican man with glioblastoma multiforme (GBM) status post two resections, complicated by hemiplegia, dysphagia, functional decline, as well as recent altered mental status, a pressure injury, seizures, and respiratory failure. During a recent family meeting, his and surrogate decision maker, Estrella, decide to pursue comfort-focused care which was consistent with Mr. Cruz's previously expressed wishes. He has been transferred to an inpatient palliative care unit (IPCU) with a plan to transition home with hospice services if safe to do so. Later in the evening, when his daughter, Yvette, arrives at the IPCU, she disagrees with the plan and asks to speak with the attending physician about changing the plan of care.

The next morning, the bedside nurse expresses concern to the IPCU attending during interprofessional team (IPT) rounds. She worries about Yvette's desire for goal non-concordant care and her use of threatening, litigious language towards staff. The IPCU attending feels overwhelmed by the number of incoming transfers to the unit and requests the IPCU social worker (SW) and chaplain meet with the family. Yvette immediately demands the SW and chaplain leave and not return unless a physician accompanies them. The chaplain and SW leave the encounter feeling deflated and underappreciated because of the lack of understanding for their roles. They are also frustrated because they were sent into a volatile situation without sufficient background information or support. When the SW and chaplain join the rounding team, they explain the daughter was irritated that a physician did not accompany them. The IPCU physician states, "Why am I the only one doing my job around here?" and leaves rounds without informing the rest of the team. You are a learner on the palliative care (PC) team, starting coverage on the IPCU this week.

What do you do now?

DISCUSSION

What is actually going on here? In summary, you have a palliative care team exhibiting signs of maladaptation due to distress and conflict. Several potential sources of these negative dynamics and dysfunction include: moral distress, suboptimal communication, and mistrust. The IPCU SW and chaplain feel devalued. The registered nurse (RN) experiences distress over being asked to provide a plan of care discordant from the patient's reported values and expectations. The IPCU attending physician experiences stress and overwhelm and the fear of a litigious family member. You, the learner, are unsure of how to proceed.

As a team, no one is effectively communicating their individual experiences of distress, nor have they explicitly verbalized a common goal or collective team priority. Instead, each team member feels either disrespected, unsupported, undervalued or excluded in the collective team. This sublimation of distress erodes each member's ability to trust and hold confidence in one another. The result is interprofessional conflict that negatively impacts patient care.

Like any clinical problem, the first step is assessment and identification of the source(s) of conflict. Conflict within a team can be grouped into three main areas: individual, interpersonal, and organizational.[1] Elements that can interfere with interpersonal communication include personality archetypes, communication styles, and power imbalances.[2] Ineffective management and role ambiguity obscure responsibility and agency within the team and fuel conflict.

Conflict is an anticipated element of teamwork, especially within a team composed of members from different disciplines who have varying goals, values, and perspectives.[3] When well managed, conflict may be generative, leading to stronger team relationships and learning opportunities that carry forward to the next challenge. When poorly managed, conflict can have negative effects on teamwork, which in turn adversely impact patient safety and outcomes, patient perceptions of the IPT, and staff satisfaction.[3,4]

At the individual level, each team member brings educational expertise and experiences that shape their values. Sexual orientation, gender identity and expression, racial identity, skin color, ethnicity, and religious or spiritual beliefs contribute to team member perspectives.[3] Each team member's positionality may impact transference, countertransference, (mis)communication, and understanding of the social contexts and communication styles of colleagues, patients, and their families. A team member's confidence or self-esteem, along with physical and mental health, may influence how they manage conflict.

Team members have varying skill in conflict management or negotiation as well as competencies in working within interprofessional teams. Some clinicians may be new to the intensity of palliative teamwork, specifically in how transference and countertransference influence their own personal responses to conflict. Moreover, the context of both patient communication and intra-team communication occurs across various power differentials. Power gradients affect which team member's goal is prioritized and overall team effectiveness, impacting trust and respect between team members.[1]

On an interpersonal level, conflict may stem from racism, sexism, and other forms of prejudice and discrimination, leading to dehumanization and disrespect. Each of the core palliative care professions (e.g., medicine, nursing, social work, chaplaincy, and pharmacy) carry their own histories of institutionalized racism, sexism, and inequity. Professional health care education often occurs within a profession-specific silo; historically, opportunities to learn collaboration and communication across disciplines have been limited.

Although both the value and importance of interprofessional teams have advanced and slow progress of changes within the medical culture has occurred, a hierarchy still exists among the clinical professions. Institutionalized values of objectivity, expertise, and hierarchy are coded with gendered and racialized histories of health care professional education. In many teams, physicians often hold an authoritative position. Other team members may fear voicing opinions due to lack of empowerment or retaliation. In environments in which interpersonal communication challenges escalate to bullying or harassment, the corresponding degradation of trust holds a lasting impact carried into future teamwork.[2] Communication may also be adversely impacted by the aforementioned medical hierarchy due to team or family members placing less value on the role of nonphysician disciplines, as in the case scenario.

Organizational culture often lacks clarity regarding profession-specific scope of practice. When added to the absence of clear institutional policies, and limitations in resources such as staffing, time, and finances, conflict may ensue.[1] Within the team structure, roles without defined boundaries contribute to conflict, especially when there is significant overlap and variability in the understanding of the team member's role, education, or scope of practice from administration, other clinicians, patients, or family members. This overlap or misunderstanding can lead to underutilization or inappropriate delegation of tasks, decreased job satisfaction, and increased turnover among staff.[1] Finally, the way a team approaches conflict can have a significant impact in whether or not the experience will be *constructive* and lead to positive improvements in communication and teamwork or *destructive* and threaten the future collaboration between team members.[1] Effective conflict resolution recognizes disagreement and fosters a culture in which disagreement is viewed not as a failure but, rather, as an inevitability and possibility for growth.

EFFECTIVE TEAMS AND CONFLICT MANAGEMENT

Whereas PC clinicians are often experts in communication skills, including listening, assessing, and navigating difficult conversations, a common misconception is that palliative care teams are expert at team management, team conflict, and team communication. However, as previously stated, conflict is inevitable in *all* teams and requires a patient and practiced approach, as well as the support of all team members. Effective teams have established psychological safety—an environment in which disagreement is met with respect, accountability, and practiced communication skills— as well as ground rules for routine communication and for navigation of intra-team conflict.[5] A myriad of models highlight the importance of shared vision, collective understanding of role, and aligned care plan goals in an environment that promotes open communication and conflict resolution. Best practice requires the IPT to consider the ways in which each team member's identities and intersectional experiences of culture, race, gender, class, and education inform their expression, communication, and approach to conflict.

The IPT is essential to modern health care delivery, incorporating the skills and knowledge of a variety of professionals to deliver optimal care to the patient. An effective IPT is imperative to the provision of excellent care, and many national organizations have studied and developed recommendations on how to develop and maintain high-functioning teams.[5] Effective teams enhance team member satisfaction; optimize patient and family experiences of care; and reduce errors through having a robust ability to identify, collaborate, and resolve external and internal communication issues.[2] IPTs benefit from shared leadership models that invite each team member to step into the role of the leader when necessary so any member of the team can initiate a dialogue regarding the need for conflict resolution.[5]

CONFLICT RESOLUTION

It is imperative that the team engage in conflict resolution to create a unified plan going forward. Various formal models exist to impart a road map for conflict. The breadth and depth of these models exceed this chapter's capacity. In Box 22.1, steps of the TeamSTEPPS DESC model are highlighted to serve as an example of how to apply a model to one area of conflict in the presented scenario.[6,7] The Further Reading section provides references for those searching for a model that best fits their team. The cultural context and who comprises the team play an integral role in the conflict model selection process.

The DESC model focuses on the conflict rather than the individual behind the conflict. In the DESC model, the team member experiencing the

---

BOX 22.1 **DESC Script: A Constructive Approach for Managing and Resolving Conflict[7]**

D—Describe the specific situation or behavior; provide concrete data.
E—Express how the situation makes you feel/what your concerns are.
S—Suggest other alternatives and seek agreement.
C—Consequences should be stated in terms of impact on established team goals; strive for consensus.

---

conflict needs to describe (*D*) what is happening. The SW could start by stating to the IPCU attending, "This morning, the chaplain and I were sent into a potentially volatile situation in which a physician had been requested, and your response was hurtful." The *E* in the DESC model instructs the clinician to express concerns regarding the conflict.

The SW shares, "I feel set up and undervalued, and this has happened before. When my role is not respected, I don't feel like an important member of this team." A positive reflective statement from the IPCU physician such as "What I'm hearing you say is you felt disrespected and undervalued, is that accurate?" can assist with aligning understanding and allowing team members to feel heard. Awareness of one's own feelings and defenses can bolster a reflective conflict resolution process. For example, the IPCU attending physician may recognize that a feeling of avoidance fueled the request of the chaplain and SW to visit the daughter. Similarly, the chaplain and SW may be experiencing countertransference of the frustration and anger from the daughter. After developing a shared understanding of the problem(s), the clinician can suggest (*S*) solutions and work with team members to develop a plan that either bridges multiple goals or identifies trade-offs of prioritizing one goal over others.[5] The SW suggests that prior to visits with patients and families, the IPCU physician provide important background information about the family dynamics and the purpose of a requested visit to clarify if they are the appropriate team member to address the issue. Additionally, the SW suggests that the they perform joint visits together if they expect conflict or significant family distress, to support one another as a team.

The final step of this model clarifies the mutually agreed upon consequence (*C*) or outcome of the plan. The SW states, "I love working here, and I would like all of us to feel comfortable setting appropriate boundaries so that we can continue to function as an effective team and provide excellent patient care." If the team is unable to internally resolve the conflict, it would be reasonable to consider other resources, such as involving a supervisor or mentor outside the department who can provide guidance and facilitate resolution.

- Maladaptive team dynamics result in dysfunction and conflict within a palliative care team.
- Palliative care teams are not immune to challenging team dynamics or power imbalances; rather they mirror existing societal inequities.
- Ineffective teams often miscommunicate and poorly negotiate conflict, which negatively impacts patient care and outcomes.
- Conflict within patient care is inevitable, particularly when team members have conflicting priorities or patients and families have differing goals of care.
- Establishing individual team-based guidelines for conflict resolution is essential for effective teamwork and patient care.

References

1. Kim S, Bochatay N, Relyea-Chew A, et al. Individual, interpersonal, and organisational factors of healthcare conflict: A scoping review. *J Interprof Care*. 2017;31(3):282–290. doi:10.1080/13561820.2016.1272558
2. Schilling S, Armaou M, Morrison Z, Carding P, Bricknell M, Connelly V. Understanding teamwork in rapidly deployed interprofessional teams in intensive and acute care: A systematic review of reviews. *PLoS One*. 2022;17(8):e0272942. doi:10.1371/journal.pone.0272942
3. Broukhim M, Yuen F, McDermott H, et al. Interprofessional conflict and conflict management in an educational setting. *Med Teach*. 2019;41(4):408–416. doi:10.1080/0142159X.2018.1480753
4. Didier A, Dzemaili S, Perrenoud B, et al. Patients' perspectives on interprofessional collaboration between health care professionals during hospitalization: A qualitative systematic review. *JBI Evid Synth*. 2020;18(6):1208–1270. doi:10.11124/JBISRIR-D-19-00121
5. Zajac S, Woods A, Tannenbaum S, Salas E, Holladay CL. Overcoming challenges to teamwork in healthcare: A team effectiveness framework and evidence-based guidance. *Front Commun*. 2021;6:606445. doi:10.3389/fcomm.2021.606445
6. Chen AS, Yau B, Revere L, Swails J. Implementation, evaluation, and outcome of TeamSTEPPS in interprofessional education: A scoping review. *J Interprof Care*. 2019;33(6):795–804. doi:10.1080/13561820.2019.1594729
7. Agency for Healthcare Research and Quality. Pocket guide: TeamSTEPPS. Updated January 2020. Accessed September 16, 2024. https://www.ahrq.gov/teamstepps/instructor/essentials/pocketguide.html

Further Reading

Altillio T, Dahlin C, Remke SS, Tucker R, Weissman D. Strategies for maximizing the health/function of palliative care teams: A resource monograph. Center to Advance Palliative Care. 2014. Accessed September 16, 2024. https://www.capc.org/documents/download/98.

Fernando G, Hughes S. Team approaches in palliative care: A review of the literature. *Int J Palliat Nurs*. 2019;25(9):444–451. doi:10.12968/ijpn.2019.25.9.444

Interprofessional Education Collaborative. Core competencies for interprofessional collaborative practice: Version 3. 2023. Accessed September 16, 2024. https://www.ipecollaborative.org/ipec-core-competencies

James TA. Teamwork as a core value in health care. Harvard Medical School. August 6, 2021. Accessed September 16, 2024. https://postgraduateeducation.hms.harvard.edu/trends-medicine/teamwork-core-value-health-care

Silverman E, Johnson S, Hudnall J, Kelly A, Shumway C. They said what!? Navigating conflict with colleagues across specialties (ODS4). *J Pain Symptom Manage*. 2022;63(5):844. doi:10.1016/j.jpainsymman.2022.02.324

23 Allocation of Scarce Resources

Justin Price

A 35-year-old patient, whose only health issue was obesity, was dying in the intensive care unit (ICU) from respiratory failure from COVID-19. The fraction of inspired oxygen was increased to 100%, and all standard treatments for COVID-19 had become ineffective. During a family meeting, the patient's sister asked, "Is there anything else that can be done?" The only viable option was an advanced therapy called extracorporeal membrane oxygenation (ECMO). At the same time, there was a 75-year-old patient with multiple comorbidities who was COVID-19 positive and suffered severe respiratory failure and also needed ECMO.

What do you do now?

DISCUSSION

As the health crisis posed by the COVID-19 pandemic continued, it was clear that the health needs in the United States far exceeded the capacity of its hospitals. This included medical equipment, supplies, and health care workers. More access was needed for artificial life support therapies such as mechanical ventilation and advanced therapies such as ECMO, which, at the time, were considered life-saving therapies.[1] The provision of ventilatory support during the COVID-19 pandemic was a complication that tested the ethics of health care systems. Health care systems and administrators were faced with critical decisions about how best to distribute care with limited resources. Now that we are beyond the COVID-19 pandemic, what strategies and protocols exist that can help us take care of our patients?

Resource allocation protocols can help streamline decision-making when prioritizing the distribution of resources. One way would be to prioritize the number of life-years saved and not the greatest good for the greatest number of people. Those who have more life-years, or more stages to pass through life, should receive the resources first. For example, with regard to ventilator support, care for those in the ICU whose life-years are reduced is withdrawn to allow for others who have more life-years to utilize those resources. Under this protocol, all patients who meet usual medical indications for ICU beds and ventilators are assigned a priority score for likelihood of survival. Patients who need ventilator support are rated a priority score of 1–8, with higher scores reflecting patients with greater need.[2] Priority scores are based on likelihood to survive the hospital course with an objective measure of acute illness severity.[2] This allocation model has been adopted by states such as Pennsylvania and New Jersey.[3] Higher priority is given to those who have a likelihood of achieving longer term survival based on the presence or absence of comorbid conditions that will influence survival.

An important consideration in determining resource allocation during the pandemic was the American Medical Association's (AMA) guidelines. The AMA recommends that health care providers be dedicated to protect the interest of their patients and this dedication should be at the forefront of allocation policies. The AMA recommends that allocation policies include the medical need, urgency of need, likelihood and anticipated duration of benefit, and effect on quality of life. According to this guideline/recommendation, the first priority should be given to patients for whom treatment will avoid premature death or extremely poor outcomes. The next priority should be patients who will experience the greatest change in quality of life. The AMA recommends using an objective, flexible, and transparent mechanism to determine which patients will receive the resources and to explain the policies and procedures to patients who are denied access to the scarce resources.

Another strategy is to create an algorithm for distributing resources. This algorithm should have an objective scoring system in place that takes into account patient acuity and meaningful survivability. To reduce bias, a health care provider who is not caring for the patient should be applying this scoring system and algorithm. This algorithm can apply to any scarce resources—that is, not just ventilators but also vaccines, therapeutics, high-flow oxygen, and oxygen tanks. Ezekiel Emanuel is the current Vice Provost for Global Initiatives at the University of Pennsylvania and Chair of the Department of Medical Ethics and Health Policy. He recommends four fundamental values for allocating scarce resources. First, maximize the benefits produced by scarce resources. Next, treat people equally, promote and reward instrumental value, and give priority to the worst off.[4] He supports the strategy of saving the most life-years by giving priority to patients likely to survive longest after treatment. He promotes treating people equally, but not on a first-come, first-served basis, and considering random selection when determining who to treat among patients with similar prognoses.

One of the challenges the United States faces is how to allocate its resources more efficiently to improve the health of the entire population. The National Academies of Sciences, Engineering, and Medicine suggests that efficient health care provides the greatest value. For example, failure to provide care that is known to be effective leads to lost opportunities. The failure to provide low-cost interventions that have well-documented efficacy and effectiveness reflects the inefficiency of the system. For example, childhood immunizations, adequate prenatal care, and appropriate screening for early diagnosis of cervical cancer are low-cost interventions with significant health benefit. Given an equal clinical outcome, expenditures should be focused on resources that are lower cost for the consumer. The National Academies suggests use of a "field model" in which the focus is moved from individual patients or a specific population to the community as a whole. The stakeholders are members of a community who review potential indicators of inefficient allocation of health care resources.

A hospital triage committee is a resource that can help create policies on how to distribute resources for a health care system.[5] A hospital triage committee can consist of respected clinicians and leaders of the health care community who are not providing direct care to patients. This allows for physicians and nurses caring for the patients to maintain their traditional roles as fiduciary advocates, and it creates the opportunity for physicians and nurses to appeal a decision from the committee. The policies from a triage committee can help with distribution of resources such as ventilatory support and ECMO treatment and important staffing issues. In addition, a triage committee can create standards that address racial and ethnic disparities, which were prominent during the COVID-19 pandemic.[6]

Health care providers do not need to make decision alone. In addition to referring to protocols and committees, a health care provider can seek assistance from other specialists to help with medical decision-making, including respiratory therapists, speech pathologists, social workers, hospital administrators, and case managers. Health care providers must acknowledge their own limitations and be open and willing to involve other health care team members.

The policies implemented for resource allocation must be ethical and guided by principles such as the Hippocratic Oath, in which treatment is provided that is beneficial and does not cause harm or hurt. The principles of beneficence, nonmaleficence, and justice are critical to any guidelines to allocate resources.[7] Beneficence is the principle of doing good and can be applied to care rationing.[8] Nonmaleficence is the principle of avoiding harm and relates to the directive *primum non nocere*—that is "first, do no harm."[9] Justice and fairness are the equitable allocation of resources and fairness in distribution of care.[2] There are times when certain groups of people should receive higher priority. As such, health care workers, first responders, and those who have a special role in the hospital or community who are critical to the effort should receive higher priority. When possible, use objective data and clinical judgment to decide the potential life-years for patients.

CASE RESOLUTION

The 35-year-old patient was dying from COVID and needed ECMO but, due to limited resources, was unable to receive it. She died; however, the 75-year-old patient with COVID did receive ECMO and remained in the hospital for more than a year and eventually died in the hospital. When you take into consideration the low likelihood of a meaningful recovery and the eventual outcome, should ECMO have been provided for the 35-year-old patient instead of the 75-year-old patient? Was the resource allocated appropriately in this case?

As outlined in this chapter, allocation policies must meet the medical need and abide by ethical principles. Priority should be given to patients for whom treatment will avoid premature death or extremely poor outcomes. In the case presented in this chapter, there were concerns that because the 35-year-old patient was obese, this could lead to additional complications on ECMO, and so ECMO was provided for a different patient who was perceived to have a greater benefit. A health care system can create an algorithm for distributing resources that best fits the community it serves. This can include a scoring system that helps prioritize those who will benefit the most. In this case, an algorithm, scoring system, and involvement of a triage committee could have helped in making the best decision.

A central purpose for health care providers is to serve patients and provide the best medical care. Some patients will have a negative outcome, but the intentions must align with the principles of benevolence, nonmaleficence, justice, and fairness. Indisputably, medical expertise is important, but these principles must be at the forefront of our decision-making. Although the COVID-19 pandemic has passed, there is a need to apply the lessons learned from the challenges encountered during it to continue to improve our policies and procedures in allocating resources to meet the health needs of the communities we serve.

- Resource allocation should be prioritized for those with the most number of life-years saved.
- An algorithm with a scoring system can help guide decision-making for medical resources.
- The principles of beneficence, nonmaleficence, and justice should be a part of any resource allocation model.
- A multidisciplinary approach should be used when making complex decisions about resource allocation.

References

1. Farrell TW, Ferrante LE, Brown T, et al. AGS position statement, resource allocation strategies and age-related considerations in the COVID-19 era and beyond. *J Am Geriatric Soc.* 2020a;68(6):1136–1142.
2. Garrett JR, McNolty LA, Wolfe ID, et al. Our next pandemic ethics challenge. Allocating "normal" health care services. *Hastings Cent Rep. 2020;50*(3):79–80.
3. Ethical policies if critical care resources become scarce. *Reliasmedia.com* 2020, April 15.
4. Emanuel EJ, Persad G, Upshur R, et al. Fair allocation of scare medical resources in the time of COVID-19. *NEJM.* 2020;*328*:2049–2055.
5. Supady A, Curtis JR, Abrams D, et al. Allocating scarce intensive care resources during the COVID-19 pandemic: Practical challenges to theoretical frameworks. *Lancet.* 2021;*9*:430–443.
6. Maves RC, Downar J, Dichter JR, et al. Triage of scarce critical care resources in COVID-19 an implementation guide for regional allocation. *Chest.* 2020;158(1):212–225.
7. White DB, Katz MH, Luce JM, Lo B. Who should receive life support during a public health emergency? Using ethical principles to improve allocation decisions. *Ann Intern Med.* 2009;150(2):132–138.
8. Ho EP, Neo HY. COVID 19: Prioritise autonomy, beneficence and conversations before score, based triage. *Age Ageing.* 2021;*50*(1):11–15.
9. Gillon R. "Primum non nocere" and the principle of non-maleficence. *Br Med J (Clinical Res ED).* 1985;*291*(6488):130–131.

24 Introducing Novel Treatments and Navigating Institutional Policies

Jennifer Winegarden

Jerry, a 76-year-old male with metastatic carcinoid and renal cell cancer involving the spinal cord, presented to a community hospital ED with intractable pain and aggressive behavior. This occurred shortly after discharge from a tertiary hospital, where he had received treatment for multiple complications, including Staphylococcus aureus urolithiasis, sepsis, osteomyelitis, and bilateral psoas abscesses. Persistent pain and psychiatric illness had significantly complicated his care. After continued medical decline, Jerry was discharged home with hospice services.

At home, Jerry experienced extreme agitation, making threats and attempts at physical violence, leading to his return to the hospital under protective services. During the palliative care team's evaluation, Jerry reported two months of severe, neuropathic pain (10/10) in the lower extremities, consistent with central sensitization. His prior pain regimen, including oxycodone, gabapentin, lidocaine patches, and quetiapine, had failed to control his symptoms.

In the ED, Jerry received IV ketamine (0.2 mg/kg), which led to marked pain relief (reduced from "10/10" to "6/10" within 45 minutes) and allowed for rest and cooperation with further evaluation. A plan was developed for low-dose IV ketamine boluses every 6 hours and opioid rotation to address central pain syndrome and potential opioid-induced hyperalgesia. However, its implementation faced resistance on the general medical floor due to safety concerns.

To address these challenges, Jerry was admitted to hospice at a general inpatient level, with education provided to the staff. However, at shift change, there was again a barrier to understanding the goals and safety of ketamine, and it was held by the nurse and a provider taking over nocturnal care. This led to a pain crisis and severe, recurrent agitation.

What do you do now?

DISCUSSION

> Experience teaches that men are often so much governed by what they are accustomed to see and practice, that the simplest and most obvious improvements . . . are adopted with hesitation, reluctance, and slow gradations.
>
> —Alexander Hamilton[1]

The evolution of medical practice frequently encounters inertia, as practitioners often adhere to established routines, resulting in reluctance to adopt even the most straightforward innovations. As articulated by Hamilton, the transition toward novel treatment modalities is typically characterized by gradual acceptance, overshadowed by prevailing customs.

In the context of palliative care, the introduction of novel therapies can instill hope in patients facing debilitating illnesses. An essential component of care involves educating patients about these advancements, thereby fostering a robust doctor-patient relationship. This educational approach is crucial for developing patient-centered treatment plans amid the complexities of increasing illness burdens. However, the introduction of new therapeutic options frequently meets resistance due to various factors, a phenomenon persisting even in an era of technological advancement and abundant educational resources.

Despite the proliferation of evidence-based guidelines, statistics indicate that "in United States healthcare delivery organizations, 40% of patients do not receive evidence-based care, ~25% of patients are harmed, and at least 30% of annual healthcare spending is wasted."[2] This highlights a significant disconnect between the availability of innovative treatment strategies and their practical implementation in clinical settings.

The latency between the introduction of innovative concepts and their integration into clinical practice remains a substantial challenge, though it may not conform to the oft-cited 17 year paradigm.[2-4] These delays have been well studied, and one initial finding is that physicians, in particular, can be slow to adapt to change. This phenomenon can be attributed to several factors including the pace at which new information disseminates, the inertia associated with prior methodologies, and the apprehension surrounding the integration of new practices into existing care paradigms.

Physicians often grapple with a fundamental shift from a focus on bio-logic plausibility—such as the assumption that monitoring blood glucose or conducting cancer screenings yields improved outcomes—to a reliance on population-based data that substantiate the efficacy of specific interventions across broader patient demographics. [4] Finally, physicians may be wary of change due to the complexity of implementing new therapies within their patient population, prior (negative) experiences of the physician, and align-ment with medical systems that hold a diminished role of education and innovation.[2]

To effect meaningful change in clinical environments, both clinicians and organizational leaders must engage in the dual process of learning and unlearning. To do so, they need to "unlearn" the old knowledge, a process that can be more difficult and lengthier than that of the learning stage. Unlearning is "the process by which individuals and organizations acknowledge and release prior learning (including assumptions and mental frameworks) in order to incorporate new information and behaviors."[3] The unlearning process involves classical evidence, personal clinical experi-ence, frequent reminders toward change, and conversations with respected colleagues. This complex process threatens a physician's "equilibrium" in practice until they not only unlearn the previously held knowledge but also work through contextual issues with the new knowledge. All this must occur while they simultaneously balance patient resistance and patient autonomy.

Some programs, such as one at Northwestern University, are engaged in designing real-world applications to provide "optimized interventions [that] could help increase adoption of best practices in hospitals around the country and increase quality of care."[5] With a similar goal, the American Academy of Hospice and Palliative Medicine published a new edition of its *Clinical Practice Guidelines for Quality Palliative Care*. A release statement regarding this work declared,

> We are in the midst of a revolution in quality measurement and ac-countability for the care and experiences of people living with serious illness, and these updated clinical practice guidelines can provide a framework to support national initiatives toward this aim.[6]

Although there is a variance with which different medical systems adapt more quickly to new practices, ground-level problems are central to all delays. In the case scenario above, treatment options differed between the large, tertiary hospital and its related community hospital. The first utilizes inpatient acute and/or chronic IV ketamine for pain consistent with the guidelines published in 2018.[7] However, no provider opted to initiate this treatment although they had the ability to deliver the medication swiftly. The smaller, but related, community hospital was inexperienced with this treatment, expressed concerns, and allowed for treatment only with stipulations. Even with these in place, some staff struggled with the treatment and even interfered with its delivery at one time. These issues are not uncommon in American medical practice.

Such differences are multifactorial but generally relate to the overall educational processes engaged by the institutions. The large hospital engages in practices that routinely provide for high-level care. Its size allows for extensive training, and therefore versatility, of its medical team. It has a depth of rapid-response support clinicians with 24-hour specialists in-house. If one practitioner—for instance, the nurse on the floor responsible for the delivery of the medication—had questions or concerns, there would likely be several other clinicians from which she could seek assistance.

These large-site academic programs have an inherent bandwidth for education and mentorship that allow for a high-level commitment to innovation. However, it takes intentional training, and a reliable level of staffing, to provide the advanced levels of care consistently in any sized setting. Addressing such gaps requires "healthcare delivery organizations [to] acquire workforces with competency in designing, implementing, and diffusing evidence-based healthcare solutions."[2] Although difficult for smaller or rural institutions, the gap between levels of care must continue to be addressed to allow for application of best practices.

Reasons for concern regarding gaps in care exist nationwide. Medical errors are one of the leading causes of death in the United States, and the packaging and delivery of treatment are often ineffective.[8] "At the same time, the scientific community publishes more than 140 clinical trials and 80 systematic reviews every single day."[2] The breadth of this knowledge base is enormous, and incorporating it into practice requires changes and integration in technology, business models, health care stakeholders, investors/funding, accountability, and physician engagement.[8]

Of these, the physician has greatest control of their own practices, their level of engagement in education, and their ability to collaborate. Those who seek to advance novel treatments should commit to developing collegial allies who understand the treatment's concepts and the potential gain for both patients and the institution. These associates can provide much needed support and, together with institutional leaders, can help create an environment of innovation. It is the influence of esteemed colleagues within a system that can bring about clinical practice change.

Given the knowledge that influential physicians can create waves of change, the researchers at Northwestern University developed a communication model for increasing the speed with which innovations are adopted. These interventions simulate the actions of a respected colleague. Some of this is based on the "catch" theory, in which physicians were observed to follow the example of one physician who modeled change. However, greater effectiveness was observed with esteemed colleague persuasion, where the respected physician provided education that is "opinionated but not too bossy."[3] Furthermore, they found that practice change reminders, occurring every 5–7 days, are very effective in implementing change, with new information being presented as a suggestion rather than an order.[3] Their focus on educational aids to the physician, in a "curbside consult" type of teaching, provided the greatest level of persuasion in the implementation of new therapies. Weiss et al. states,

A hospital's physicians determine whether a new diagnostic method is adopted or not. In these and many other cases, there is clear societal interest in harnessing social networks to accelerate the adoption of the best practices and the obsolescence of poor practices.[9]

Whatever methods are engaged for the introduction of novel treatments, those who are committed to see their success will need to develop a deep level of tenacity. This depth of dedication has been exemplified by Joseph Lister's commitment to handwashing and, more recently, that of Professor Graeme Clark in developing the cochlear implant. Clark recounts facing difficulties on many fronts.[6] He states,

I had much criticism and was referred to as "that clown Clark." But I was determined to persist and see it through, and I'm so pleased

I did. I cannot imagine any technology that has had such a profound effect on transforming so many peoples' lives.[10,11]

Developing an environment of innovation relies on continued education with peers and institutional leaders, collegial relationships, regular practice reminders, and intentional engagement in the learning and unlearning process. Successful innovation requires a commitment to evidence-based practice and a tolerance to tensions between evidence and context. Whether attempting to change clinical practice with already published data or introducing original treatment ideas, challenges may be overcome with communication, education, positive data, and persistence toward best practices. While waiting for corroboration with colleagues and institutional leaders, one can be providing lectures on the topic, publishing papers that report responses to the treatment (even case studies or series), and attending related seminars.

The following are steps to innovation with a novel treatment:

1. Prepare a scope of treatment, cost analysis, and potential adverse effects of treatment.
2. Present the treatment to your supervising department chair/administration as a viable option; provide data, papers, and so on.
3. Provide education on the topic to medical groups when possible.
4. Find an influential, supporting colleague and leverage their support and involvement within your medical system.
5. Educate your patient toward treatment options, but do not incriminate the institution.
6. If your treatment has been utilized, keep an updated list of data: patients treated, response, and cost. The retrospective analysis of effectiveness, practicality, and adverse events could help determine future generalizability.
7. Continue to educate yourself on the topic by reading related research topics, attending conferences, and reaching out to other physicians utilizing the treatment.
8. Don't give up.

Aligning oneself with other like-minded physicians can be a strength to one's practice goals as well as provide a foundation for institutional change.

An example of this was the founding principles displayed by Dr. William W. Mayo, who established the Mayo Clinic with his two physician sons. They dedicated a portion of each year to obtaining leading medical practices from throughout the world, incorporating them into patient care, and teaching others to do the same.

Those, like the Doctors Mayo, who advance medical practice, even within the otherwise small confines of a solitary practice, can forever change the landscape of medicine. Dr. William J. Mayo stated in 1910, "The best interest of the patient is the only interest to be considered, and in order that the sick may have the benefit of advancing knowledge, union of forces is necessary." In 1929, 10 years before his death, he stated, "I look through a half-opened door into the future, full of interest, intriguing beyond my power to describe."[12]

CASE RESOLUTION

Although Jerry's IV ketamine was withheld one evening, the staff responsible for this received education, and the medication was restarted the next day. Shortly after, pain was controlled, and this reduced his agitation. The patient remained under hospice general inpatient (GIP) care for 14 days. During that time, Jerry had many days of being alert, talking with family, and eating his favorite foods. He died peacefully with his symptoms under good control.

The institutional challenges to the use of IV ketamine on the general medical floor were related to the lack of facility experience and education. The initial concerns regarding IV ketamine were overcome by education to involved departments and the involvement of hospital pharmacists and administration. The hospital developed a ketamine order set which became utilized in all units with success.

Further collaboration and education occurred between the palliative medicine departments of the two facilities. Detailed review of the case resulted in discussion of how the treatment, discharge, and subsequent readmission for GIP hospice care could have proceeded more smoothly. Barriers to treatment and care were discussed, which benefited both departments.

- Attempting practice change with a novel treatment is not an idle process. One should be engaged in a number of steps toward implementation.
- Creating an environment of innovation requires commitment to research, the learning and unlearning process, and forging collegial relationships within the institution.
- It is a medical system's physicians that determine the adoption of best practices. Form a team of like-minded individuals who can help engage medical and administrative stakeholders.

References

1. Inspiring Quotes. n.d. Accessed January 12, 2022. https://www.inspiringquotes. us/quotes/9VNr_LClmena0
2. Mehta J, Aalsma MC, O'Brien A, et al. Becoming an agile change conductor. *Front Public Health*. 2022;10:1044702. doi:10.3389/fpubh.2022.1044702
3. Gupta DM, Boland RJ, Aron DC. The physician's experience of changing clinical practice: A struggle to unlearn. *Implement Sci*. 2017; 12:28.
4. Ebell MH, Shaughnessy AF, Slawson DC. Why are we so slow to adopt some evidence-based practices? *Am Fam Physician*. 2018;98(12):709–710.
5. Northwestern University. Persuading doctors to quickly adopt new treatments. *Science Daily*. October 27, 2014.
6. Rotella J, Twaddle ML. New national quality guidelines keep pace with rapid advances in palliative care. American Academy of Hospice and Palliative Medicine. n.d. Accessed October 12, 2022. https://aahpm.org/quarterly/winter-18-feature
7. Schwenk ES, Viscusi ER, Buvanendran A, et al. Consensus guidelines on the use of intravenous ketamine infusions for acute pain management from the American Society of Regional Anesthesia and Pain Medicine, the American Academy of Pain Medicine, and the American Society of Anesthesiologists. *Reg Anesth Pain Med*. 2018;43(5):456–466. doi:10.1097/AAP.0000000000000806
8. Herzlinger RE. Why innovation in health care is so hard. *Harv Bus Rev*. 2006;84(5):58–66, 156. https://pubmed.ncbi.nlm.nih.gov/16649698
9. Weiss CH, Poncela-Casasnovas J, Glaser JI, et al. Adoption of a high-impact innovation in a homogeneous population. *Phys Rev X*. 2014;4(4):041008.
10. Marsh, A. The long road to today's cochlear implant: Graeme Clark's dogged pursuit of the technology enabled hundreds of thousands of people to hear. *IEEE Spectrum*. January 27, 2022. https://spectrum.ieee.org/cochlear-implant-history.

11. Wikipedia contributors. Graeme Clark (doctor). Wikipedia. November 19, 2022. Accessed October 2, 2022. https://en.wikipedia.org/w/index.php?title=Graeme_Clark_(doctor)&oldid=1122719948

12. Mayo Clinic. History & heritage: Quotations from the Doctors Mayo. n.d. Accessed December 1, 2023. https://history.mayoclinic.org/toolkit/quotations/the-doctors-mayo.php

25 Racial Inequities in Health Care

Carmen Renee Green

A 64-year-old African American man with chronic thoracolumbar back pain relocated to a nearby community and presents to a large Midwestern academic pain center. He was previously treated at a large Northeastern academic pain center for failed back pain due to epidural fibrosis, arachnoiditis, and spinal cord stenosis. He is disabled, and his pain has been managed with morphine 90 mg p.o. t.i.d., gabapentin 900 mg p.o. t.i.d., and acetaminophen 650 mg p.o. t.i.d. for 15 years. He also has a spinal cord stimulator and reports a pain score of 7/10 at worst and 5/10 at best. He states that his pain never goes away, his sleep is interrupted, and his mood is "okay." He wishes to continue his current pain management regimen, which helps him maintain some semblance of quality of life. What he needs is a new doctor to manage his pain regimen and states, "If necessary, I will participate in random drug screening and pill counts."

What do you do now?

DISCUSSION

Central to optimizing the health care experience and patient satisfaction is high-quality bidirectional communication between the person with the disease and their clinician. Ideally, a complete family, social, medical, and surgical history is obtained, and a focused physical exam is performed. Together, these components should drive clinician decision-making in a patient-centered manner. However, the process is also influenced by human factors such as the condition being assessed and treated; clinician and patient attitudes; and patient and clinician race, ethnicity, gender, and class (and other social determinants of health).[1-4] It is important to note that physicians are often in the top quintile of income earners, and the percentage of Black physicians (~5%) in the United States has remained less than their representation in society (~13.9%) for several decades.

Regardless of socioeconomic status, minoritized patients are at significant risk for suboptimal health care regardless of the health condition being assessed, including those for which Black people have an increased prevalence compared to Whites.[3-5] This is especially true when Black people seek and receive pain care.[1-3] Clinician decision-making further varies based on the type of pain (acute, chronic, and cancer), further complicating access to pain care and the quality of care.[5] Clinicians consistently have lower goals for chronic pain management compared to acute and cancer pain management, and they are increasingly reluctant to prescribe opioids for all types of pain.[6]

Race is a social construct based on phenotype and is intrinsically related to economic power.[7-9] In the case of Black race, it is often associated with conscious, unconscious, and implicit bias as well as negative stereotypes and false narratives that negatively influence the quality of health and pain care.[1] During the clinical interaction, it is important to go beyond obtaining a generic history and performing a physical exam to get a fundamental understanding of the patient's history, lived experience, and ecosystem. When considering a societal and historical lens, it is important to note that pain was used to control behavior and to inflict fear.[10] Both the fact that Black people were chattel slaves and the fact that race-based discrimination was used to perpetuate their enslavement and to sanction ongoing segregation and experimentation following their emancipation have yielded profound trust issues that continue to complicate their care and their willingness to participate in research studies. In addition to White slave owners, scientists and clinicians alike championed experimenting on enslaved and free Black people. These actions and attitudes have long-standing repercussions that haunt us today.

Several studies show that Black people have diminished access to care and are more likely not to have their pain appropriately assessed, to receive lesser quality care for similar conditions, and to have worse health outcomes compared to Whites.[3] A study revealed that Black patients and their visitors were more than twice as likely to have hospital security called on them than White patients and their visitors.[10] Another study showed that White medical students and residents had similar beliefs about biological differences between Black and White people, similar to some of their forefathers, which predicted race-based bias in pain perception contributing to poor treatment recommendations for Black people.[11] Complicating false physiological, biological, and innate beliefs about differences between Black and White people are a pedagogy and attitudes supporting an increased risk for psychological conditions such as addiction, feigning disability, and propensity toward criminality among Black people. Altogether, this has prompted additional scrutiny, monitoring, and decreased access to analgesic care, further perpetuating race-based health disparities and inequities associated with worse health outcomes for Black people.[12,13]

Throughout history, false beliefs and racial bias have yielded problematic assessment and the undertreatment of chronic pain regardless of the modality (e.g., opioid analgesics and nerve blocks) in Black people, with a profound effect on their quality of life. Furthermore, concerns about substance abuse and addiction have been attributed to Black people without data to support they are at increased risk, further impairing their care.

Behavioral and social determinants (i.e., where people work, live, play, and pray) affect health and well-being. Yet, rarely are attempts made to obtain this information or fully understand the patient's complete story. In the case of Black and Brown people, their story may include long-standing and ongoing race/ethnic-based microaggressions, macroaggressions, and health care injustices that negatively impact their quality of life. To improve quality of care and quality of life will require clinicians to actively listen to stories they may find uncomfortable to hear and a willingness to understand bias to promote understanding and trust within health care.[13]

CASE RESOLUTION

Clinicians at the Midwestern academic pain center were able to obtain and review medical records and talk to the patient's prior physician, who stated, "He's a good patient, not a drug seeker." Previously, the patient was an engineer and an automobile executive for one of the Big Three auto manufacturers. His life changed when a 17-year-old drunk driver ran a red light and T-boned the car he was driving. He was unconscious and spent several weeks in critical care to treat a subdural hematoma, a pneumothorax, and multiple fractures (including ribs and long bones). Six months after his hospitalization, his low back pain persisted despite physical therapy and other modalities. He had three epidural steroid injections by an outside-the-system pain doctor. His care was complicated by osteomyelitis and multiple failed back surgeries. His pain was never managed well, and a spinal cord stimulator placed a few years later to address his radicular pain provided partial relief for 5 years. He concluded, "They did what they could" and decided to move in with his daughter and 12-year-old grandson so they could support each other.

In many ways, the rest of the patient's story is unexpected. Pain's devastating impact on quality of life and socioeconomic status is real. The presence of chronic pain generally leads to a significant reduction in quality of life and socioeconomic status. The easy thing to do is to determine that little can be done to help him; however, more can be done. There are important considerations based on his race, and socioeconomic status does not protect African American patients from variability in health care decision-making nor the injustice in the same ways it does for White patients. All people want to be heard, treated with compassion and respect, and receive high-quality equitable care that improves their quality of life such that they have more good days than bad. Thus, empathy, an open mind, and a listening ear may be more important than the clinician's stethoscope or reflex hammer in addressing racial inequities in health and pain care.

- Adopt anti-racist tenets into patient bills of rights, professional charters, and codes of conduct.
- Incorporate bias and ethics training at the organizational level.
- Use social determinants of health to address disparities.
- Audit institutional data and incorporate continuous quality improvement principles.
- Incorporate diverse voices and leadership, including potential new leaders.
- Consider implementing a truth and reconciliation process.
- Examine the legacy of pain research and care.
- Become an active listener: culturally sensitive, humble, and committed to rectifying prior harms.

Adapted from Green.[1]

References

1. Green CR. The genesis of the unequal burden of pain: A selective review examining social inequities and unheard voices. *Pain*. 2023;164(6):1258–1263.
2. Green CR, Wheeler JC, LaPorte F. Clinical decision making in pain management: Contributions of physician and patient characteristics to variations in practice. *J Pain*. 2003;4(1):29–39.
3. Green CR, Anderson KO, Baker TA, et al. The unequal burden of pain: Confronting racial and ethnic disparities in pain. *Pain Med*. 2003;4(3):277–294.
4. Marmot M: Achieving health equity: From root causes to fair outcomes. *Lancet*. 2007;370:1153–1163.
5. Green CR, Hart-Johnson T. The association between race and neighborhood socioeconomic status in younger Black and White adults with chronic pain. *J Pain*. 2012; 13(2): 176–186.
6. Green CR, Ndao-Brumblay SK, West B, Washington T. Differences in prescription opioid analgesic availability: Comparing minority and White pharmacies across Michigan. *J Pain*. 2005;6(10):689–699.
7. Baker TA, Green CR. Intrarace differences among Black and White Americans presenting for chronic pain management: The influence of age, physical health, and psychosocial factors. *Pain Med*. 2005;6(1):29–38.
8. Green CR, Ndao-Brumblay SK, Nagrant AM, Baker TA, Rothman E. Race, age, and gender influences among clusters of African American and White patients with chronic pain patients. *J Pain*. 2004;5(3):171–182.

9. Green CR, Baker TA, Smith EM, Sato Y. The effect of race in older adults presenting for chronic pain management: A comparative study of Black and White Americans. *J Pain*. 2003;4(2):82–90.

10. Green CR, McCullough WR, Hawley JD. Visiting Black patients: Racial disparities in security standby requests. *J Natl Med Assoc*. 2018;110;37–43.

11. Hoffman KM, Trawalter S, Axt JR, Oliver MN. Racial bias in pain assessment and treatment recommendations, and false beliefs about biological differences between Blacks and Whites. *Proc Natl Acad Sci USA*. 2016;113(16):4296–4301. doi:10.1073/pnas.1516047113

12. Green CR. Being present: The role of narrative medicine in reducing the unequal burden of pain. *Pain* 2011;152(2):965–966.

13. Green CR. Unequal burdens and unheard voices: Whose pain? Whose narratives? In: Carr DB, Loeser JD, Morris DB, eds. *Narrative, Pain, and Suffering* (Progress in Pain Research and Management, Vol. 34). IASP Press; 2005:195–213.

PART V

Dilemmas Related to Ethical Issues

26 Artificial Hydration and Nutrition at the End of Life

Carol Pilgrim and Tamara Vesel

XC is a 72-year-old Mandarin-speaking male with a history of advanced dementia and recurrent aspiration pneumonia. He was hospitalized with pneumonia 5 months ago and discharged on home hospice. Last night, he was readmitted after presenting to the emergency department with dyspnea. When the primary team met with the family members, they said they wanted to keep their father comfortable. The admitting team discontinued XC's intravenous (IV) fluids as part of the comfort care order set, but now the family is requesting IV hydration.

GS, a 5-day old newborn, presents to the emergency department following a home birth complicated by a placental abruption and hypoxia. He was extubated to nasal continuous positive airway pressure but is unable to swallow. His ultrasound shows diffuse axonal injury and a grade 4 bleed bilaterally. The neurologist and neonatologist meet with the family to discuss prognosis. The parents request discontinuing artificial nutrition, saying they "do not want to prolong his suffering." The neonatal intensive care unit (NICU) team is conflicted about what to do because they do not want to "hasten the newborn death."

Palliative care is frequently consulted to assist in end-of-life discussions, especially if members of the team and the family are experiencing conflict or distress. Both cases revolve around questions posed by family members or members of the health care team about the use of artificial nutrition and hydration at the end of life. Is it appropriate to administer artificial hydration to a patient who is actively dying? Is it ethical to withdraw artificial nutrition? As the clinician assigned to both these cases, you should start by performing a comprehensive assessment to better understand the source of these tensions.

Five months ago, XC was admitted for aspiration pneumonia that resulted in respiratory failure requiring mechanical ventilation. During that admission, XC had a modified barium swallow evaluation performed, which revealed silent aspiration. At that time, the family indicated that XC would not want a feeding tube, and he was discharged home with home hospice.

XC's son, who speaks English fluently, is the health care proxy. He reports that when he brought his father home following the last admission, his father initially got better. However, during the last couple of weeks his father has become increasingly confused and is now too weak to get out of bed. Two nights ago, his father suddenly became short of breath. The son called the hospice nurse, who instructed him to give his father morphine. However, a few hours later, his father's work of breathing had not stabilized, and XC's son brought him to the emergency department.

The team offered to place a nasogastric (NG) tube, but XC's son declined it because during the last admission when his father had a feeding tube, he had become agitated. XC's family agreed with the team's recommendation to stop antibiotics and focus on comfort. The medical team changed XC's code status to "comfort measures only." As part of the comfort care order set, the team discontinued the patient's maintenance fluids. The following morning, XC's family requests resuming IV fluids. This request prompts the team to consult palliative care to "explain comfort measures only to the family." The nurse, who is concerned the patient is actively dying, pages palliative care STAT to the bedside. On exam, XC is unresponsive. His mouth is dry. His breathing is irregular, and his hands and feet are mottled.

In the case of XC, the medical team's understanding of appropriate care for a patient whose code status is *comfort measures only* does not include artificial nutrition and hydration. "The order set says to discontinue IV fluids." Their view conflicts with his family's view that XC will die from dehydration unless IV fluids are resumed. Members of the nursing team are experiencing both distress and conflict. They are at the bedside fielding the family's request for IV fluids. They are uncomfortable because they recognize that XC is imminently dying while his family is not realizing that the death is imminent. They do not think that XC will benefit from fluid administration, and they wish the family would have the same understanding. XC's family members see their father opened mouth, too weak to even swallow, and fear he is suffering. They are distressed because treatments they believe would benefit their father were discontinued without their knowledge, and they are angry with both the nurses for not administering fluids and the physician in charge for not ordering them.

In the NICU, the staff differ with baby GS's parents in their evaluation of the benefits and burdens of continuing artificial nutrition through an NG tube. They worry that by discontinuing nutrition, they would be responsible for hastening the death of a neonate. They are more comfortable in a world in which high-tech interventions are used to save young life than in a world in which neonates die. The parents are sitting in unimaginable grief. They do not want to continue a treatment they believe would prolong their newborn son's suffering.

As the palliative care clinician, it is your job to facilitate communication between families and the health care team. Back et al.[1] provide a comprehensive guide for communicating with seriously ill patients and their families. They recommend the health care team pre-meet prior to a family conference. This pre-meeting allows you to find out what the clinical team already knows about the patient and their family. A pre-meeting also creates a space for the team to verbalize any concerns they might have. You learn from XC's nurse that his daughter used all her vacation time during his previous admission and is planning on going in to work. She has also brought her father soup and is upset that he is too weak to eat it. Meeting with the team taking care of GS, you learn that one of the physicians on the team believes strongly that GS's artificial nutrition should be continued.

You arrange a conference with the medical team, social work, nursing, and XC's family. After introductions, you should begin by assessing the family's understanding of the patient's medical condition.[1] This assessment should include the events leading up to admission, any underlying chronic illnesses, the hospital course, and understanding of prognosis. In addition, the clinician should explore the patient's value system and their spiritual and cultural traditions.

XC developed aspiration pneumonia in the setting of Alzheimer's dementia. Dementia is a persistent, progressive disease that results in impaired cognitive and intellectual functioning.[2] Initially, patients with dementia experience issues with memory, language, and executive function. As the disease progresses, the parts of the brain that control vital functions such as swallowing are affected, thereby putting patients such as XC at risk for aspiration. Patients with dementia commonly die from the complications of dementia (e.g., trouble swallowing, difficulty communicating with family and providers about symptoms, decreased mobility leading to infection, and injury from falls). Although it is possible to respond to each individual event, the trajectory cannot be changed.

In the case of XC, his family understands that their father has dementia and has experienced recurrent pneumonias. They confirm a feeding tube would not be within goals of care and agree that continuing antibiotics is not indicated. However, it is evident after they share their understanding of their father's illness that they do not know their father is in the *present moment dying of dementia* and focus on his being too weak to eat the soup the daughter brought and the fear he will die of thirst without IV fluids.

After assessing the family's understanding, the clinician should ask permission to provide a medical update.[1] Clinicians are often uncomfortable when faced with predicting when a patient will die. However, if you think that a patient is dying or will not recover, it is imperative to let the family know and provide anticipatory guidance. Teach the family about signs of the terminal phase of illness and the phase of dying. If the goal is comfort, this clarity also saves patients from undergoing unnecessary tests, interventions, and procedures.[3]

You should continue to perform a physical exam in patients who are approaching death.[4] An exam can reveal signs of imminent death. Look for signs such as decreased response to verbal and visual stimuli, peripheral cyanosis, respirations with mandibular movement, pooled oral secretions, inability to close eyes, Cheyne–Stokes respirations, dropping of nasolabial fold, and hyperextension of the neck.

Do not expect that patients and their families will understand that focusing on comfort equates to end-of-life care. XC's children brought him to the hospital because they did not recognize symptoms of dying in a patient with dementia. Help them place his current condition in the context of his steady decline from dementia. Reference signs and symptoms his family has already noted (confusion, recurrent infections, growing weaker, and the inability to get out of bed), and point out the signs of imminent death noted on exam.

Use simple, unambiguous language to explain that their father is dying and that he has likely hours to days. Learn to be comfortable making space for grief rather than using language that obscures it. It is difficult to use the words death and dying, but learn to use them.[1]

After sharing the assessment that XC is imminently dying, you should check in with his family and address any questions or concerns. In this case, the family discusses that after the meeting yesterday, they had understood that the patient's dementia was not treatable, but they had not understood that time was limited to hours to days. Although the family and medical team had agreed to "comfort," the family did not have a sense of timing. They did not recognize that their father was in the normal dying process, so they mistakenly attributed the change in his responsiveness to the discontinuation of IV fluids.

Use what you learned about the family and make medical recommendations based on their values and worldview.[1] Begin by talking about the care you recommend, and then move to talking about medical care you do not recommend and why. Explain how the team will continue to care for XC and help maintain his dignity until the end of his life. Discuss the use of medications to control symptoms. If appropriate, offer the support of social work and spiritual care. Let XC's family know you do not recommend restarting IV fluids and explain why. Anorexia–cachexia syndrome is part of the dying process. You should explain to family members that decreased appetite is the result of the body slowing down and preparing for death as it loses the ability to use food for energy.[3]

XC's daughter's concern about her father dying of thirst is very common. Share with the family that artificial nutrition and hydration will not prolong the life of a terminally ill patient who is actively dying.[5] Artificial hydration and nutrition are considered medical interventions, and you should discuss the potential benefits and burdens of medical interventions as part of shared decision-making.[6] The burdens of artificial hydration and nutrition include worsening agitation, infections associated with lines and tubes, aspiration, diarrhea from tube feeds, and fluid overload.[5] Recognize that bringing in food is a sign of the family's instinct to provide care and help them find alternatives. After a discussion of the burdens of artificial hydration and other measures that can be used to ensure XC's comfort, his family agrees to forgo artificial hydration in favor of less invasive ways to alleviate thirst and dry mouth, such as ice chips and excellent oral care. They understand that their father is dying of dementia and not dehydration.

Questions surrounding artificial hydration and nutrition at the end of life can be emotionally charged for patients, families, and clinicians alike. Providing food and nourishment is intrinsic to our sense of what it means to care for another. In the case of baby GS in the NICU, the baby's parents are asking to stop artificial hydration and nutrition, and members of the medical team are reluctant to stop feedings administered via NG tube. They are worried about hastening a newborn's death. The palliative care clinician's role is to support the infant as well as the baby's parents and the medical providers.

Although withdrawing a medical intervention can feel more emotionally challenging than the decision to never have started it, ethically, withdrawing a therapy is no different than making the decision initially to withhold it. Artificial hydration and nutrition are considered medical treatments, and like all medical treatments, the decision to start or discontinue a therapy should be based on the clinical circumstances.[6]

Patients', families', and health care providers' approaches to caring for a dying person map to their life experiences as well as their religious, spiritual, and cultural values and traditions.[7] You should share data about the benefits and burdens of artificial hydration and nutrition while understanding that some traditions may ascribe importance to these interventions beyond the physical. In these circumstances, you should explore these beliefs. If the family continues to hold that providing IV fluids is a moral mandate, it is reasonable to offer a limited trial of gentle hydration along with warning the family about the potential for fluid overload.[3]

Clinicians also bring their own set of values, experiences, and traditions to their work. During the pre-meeting, one of the physicians assigned to the

NICU expressed discomfort with discontinuing GS's tube feeds. A health care professional who has a clear moral or religious objection to the plan of care may not abandon a patient, but they may seek to transfer care of the patient to another provider. Many institutions have an ethics committee that can help articulate rights and obligations of the parties involved.[6]

Back in the NICU, another family meeting is held with GS's parents, neurology, and neonatology. This time they are joined by a member of the palliative care team who can address the ethics of forgoing artificial nutrition. As with adult patients, when working with a life-threatening or terminally ill child, the clinician should be open about the expected course and prognosis.[8] Likewise, a decision to forgo or withdraw life-sustaining therapies should be based on an assessment of the therapies' benefits and burdens. In cases of newborns with life-threatening illnesses, medical decision-making is based on the parent's or guardian's assessment of what is in the best interest of the child.[6]

It is your obligation to help the parents apply this "best interest" standard. GS's parents expressed that "feeds are only prolonging their son's suffering." With the support of the palliative care team, the medical team moves forward with removing GS's feeding tube and discontinuing his tube feedings.

Families often inquire how long a person can go without nutrition or hydration. A survey of hospice patients who stopped eating and drinking found that more than half of the patients died within 1 week.[9] XC, who exhibited signs of imminent death, died the following day. Baby GS survived 27 days after his NG tube was removed. His parents expressed concern regarding continued suffering. The team noted that baby GS was receiving some IV fluids as the solvent for medications used to manage symptoms and worked with the pharmacist to concentrate medications when possible.

XC and his family had expressed that one of the goals was time at home. However, because the family did not recognize the dying process, they brought him to the hospital. The team believed he was too close to death to transfer and that he may die during transport. XC died peacefully in the hospital with his family at his bedside. Understanding that her father was dying, XCs daughter applied for family medical leave so she could be by her father's side.

GS's parents opted to keep him in his "medical home" where they could benefit from the support of the hospital team. Palliative care followed for the remainder of his life—managing end-of-life symptoms and supporting the family and the medical team. Although working with patients and families to elucidate goals and develop a plan of care that aligns with those goals is fundamental to being a palliative care clinician, the work does not stop there. In both cases, palliative care remained involved to help manage end-of-life symptoms and shepherd the patient's family along the path of providing care and being present while simultaneously letting go. It is important to express to families how it has been an honor and privilege to be allowed to share these intimate moments with them.[1] Cases such as these are challenging, but they are also ultimately rewarding for all professionals involved.

KEY POINTS TO REMEMBER

- Do not assume everyone is on the same page. Make a point of asking patients, families, and other providers what they understand prior to giving information.
- Become comfortable using the words death and dying. Avoid euphemisms.
- Remember you are part of a multidisciplinary team. Involving social work, pastoral care, nursing, and ethics can help in difficult cases.
- Although artificial nutrition and hydration are medical interventions that can be stopped if the benefits do not outweigh the burden, as humans we ascribe meaning to feeding beyond the physical.

References

1. Back A, Arnold R, Tulsky J. *Mastering Communication with Seriously Ill Patients: Balancing Honesty with Empathy and Hope.* Cambridge University Press; 2009.
2. Olson E. Dementia and neurodegenerative disorders. In: Morrison RS, Meier DE, eds. *Geriatric Palliative Care.* Oxford University Press; 2003:160–172.
3. Lacey J, Cherny NI. Management of the actively dying patient. In: Cherny NI, Fallon MT, Kaasa S, Portenoy RK, Currow DC, eds. *Oxford Textbook of Palliative Medicine.* 6th ed. Oxford University Press; 2021:1104–1118.

4. Hui D, Mori M. Physiology of dying. In: Cherny NI, Fallon MT, Kaasa S, Portenoy RK, Currow DC, eds. *Oxford Textbook of Palliative Medicine*. 6th ed. Oxford University Press; 2021:1094–1103.

5. American Academy of Hospice and Palliative Medicine. Statement on artificial nutrition and hydration near the end of life. September 13, 2013. Accessed January 22, 2023. https://aahpm.org/positions/anh

6. Berlinger N, Jenning B, Wolf WM. *The Hastings Center Guidelines for Decisions on Life-Sustaining Treatment and Care Near the End of Life*. 2nd ed. Oxford University Press; 2013.

7. Blank RH. End-of-life decision making across cultures. *J Law Med Ethics*. 2011;39(2):201–214.

8. American Academy of Pediatrics. Committee on Bioethics and Committee on Hospital Care. Palliative care for children. *Pediatrics*. 2000;106(2 Pt 1):351–357.

9. Pasman HR, Onwuteaka-Philipsen BD, Kriegsman DM, Ooms ME, Ribbe MW, van der Wal G. Discomfort in nursing home patients with severe dementia in whom artificial nutrition and hydration is forgone. *Arch Intern Med*. 2005;165(15):1729–1735.

Physician-Assisted Death

Sudha Chandrasekhar

Dr. Robert Milton is a 41-year-old brilliant, fiercely independent, Nobel Laureate who has dedicated his life to science and research. Research is his religion; science is his God. He has a rare mixed small cell neuroendocrine tumor in his nasal cavity that is widely metastatic to lungs, liver, and brain. He underwent four surgeries and three rounds of aggressive chemotherapy in 11 months, including a new trial protocol. Unfortunately, he suffered a major stroke, leaving him hemiplegic, aphasic, bed-bound, and totally dependent for all care. He now has progressive multiorgan failure. He declined dialysis, intubation, and mechanical ventilation, and he was transitioned to home hospice. But he continues to experience intolerable physical and existential distress despite state-of-the art supportive care.

You are his oncologist and personal friend. You get a call from Mrs. Milton that your patient wants to see you. She tearfully hands you his note that you can barely decipher. It reads, "Dr. Jones, I am ready to die. Please help me die." Your religious, ethical, and moral convictions do not support physician-assisted death (PAD). Yet, you feel bound by your professional responsibility, and personal friendship, to help him.

What do you do now?

DISCUSSION

At the outset, it is important to understand the various terms used to describe medically aided death:

Physician-assisted death (PAD): The physician provides, at the patient's request, a prescription for a lethal dose of medication that the patient can self-administer by ingestion, with the explicit intention of ending life. Other terms for PAD include physician-assisted suicide, physician aid in dying, patient-administered physician-hastened death, self-administered medical assistance in dying, and medical aid in dying.

Voluntary active euthanasia (VAE): VAE, or simply "euthanasia," is a term used to identify the practice whereby the clinician administers a lethal medication at the patient's request, usually by intravenous push injection. *Euthanasia is not legal in the United States.*

Medical aid/assistance in dying (MAID): Originating in Canada, this term is used to refer to both PAD and VAE, replacing either or both. In the United States, MAID is synonymous with PAD (i.e., patient-administered, physician-hastened death).

In the United States, the right-to-die movement was first legalized in Oregon in 1997. It is currently legal in 10 states (California, Colorado, Hawaii, Maine, New Jersey, New Mexico, Montana, Oregon, Vermont, and Washington) and the District of Columbia, with pending legislation in an additional 20 states. The 2021 annual report of the Death with Dignity National forum states an estimated 73 million Americans (i.e., 1 in 5 Americans) now have legal access to medically assisted aid in dying. Assisted dying practices are now legal in 18 jurisdictions, with more than 200 million people globally having access to euthanasia and/or PAD. PAD is legal in Canada, Australia, and New Zealand. Euthanasia is legal in Belgium, the Netherlands, Luxembourg, Switzerland, Germany, and Spain.

Physicians who receive a request for hastened death may experience conflicting emotions such as surprise, shock, anxiety, shame, failure, and self-doubt. Regardless of one's ethical stance on PAD, physicians have an obligation to acknowledge and respond to the patient's request (Box 27.1).

BOX 27.1 **General Guidelines for Responding to PAD Request**

What is the patient really asking?

- Consider the request as a new "symptom" to be explored by detailed history-taking.
- Acknowledge and validate what the patient has verbalized.
- Use open-ended questions, such as the following:
  - "What is the most difficult part of your current situation?"
  - "What made you decide to ask for this kind of help right now?"
  - "What are you most worried about?"

What underlies the request?

- What are the patient's fears, concerns, and emotional context of the request?
- What makes their current (or future) situation so unacceptable?
- What are the root causes of the patient's suffering?

When is the patient seeking PAD?

- Is the request for immediate PAD or future hypothetical assistance?
- It is not necessary to act on the request immediately.
- Failure to acknowledge and address the request in a timely manner may heighten the patient's distress.

How do you feel about the request?

- What makes sense for this patient?
- What feels right for you?
- Can you continue to provide potentially lethal medications that the patient may use in other ways?
- What circumstances or assurances would help you continue providing potentially lethal prescription medications?
- Can you remain emotionally involved to support the patient even if you cannot accede to the request?
- Can you provide reassurance such as "How can I help you, short of ending your life, to get through this terrible time?"

What are your legal responsibilities?

- Is the patient an adult resident of a state in which such a law is in effect?
- Is the patient capable of making and communicating their own health care decisions?
- Does the patient have a terminal illness that will lead to death within 6 months, as confirmed by qualified health care providers?
- Is the patient capable of self-administering and ingesting medications without assistance?

If there are legal options for which the patient qualifies that you cannot provide for personal reasons, you are morally (although not legally) obligated to let the patient know such options are available, how to access them, and to whom the patient can transfer.

What are your practical considerations?

- Is the patient depressed and/or suicidal?
- Does the patient have decisional capacity?
- Does the patient have an advance directive and/or designated health care agent?
- Is the patient making the request voluntarily?
- Does the patient understand that exploring the request does not obligate acting on it?
- Does the patient understand that the request can be withdrawn at any time?
- Who is the second physician willing to certify the patient meets criteria for PAD?
- What is the required wait time (varies by state) after the request is made and approved?
- What are the availability, doses, and prices of lethal drugs you plan to prescribe?
- Can the patient swallow the lethal dose of 90–100 pills?

What are the potential complications of PAD?

- Patients who ingest lethal sedatives can experience burning, nausea, vomiting, and regurgitation, especially if there is difficulty swallowing large volumes of liquid.
- Pretreatment with antiemetic is needed to minimize the risk of vomiting.
- Insufficient drug absorption can rarely lead to seizures or regaining consciousness.

Are there mutually agreeable alternatives to PAD?

- Intensification of pain and symptom management involves systematic increases in potentially effective palliative treatments, especially opioids and benzodiazepines, for intractable physical symptoms.
- Stopping or not starting potentially life-sustaining therapy such as major mechanical interventions (e.g., ventilatory support, dialysis, and ventricular assist devices) and seemingly simple medicinal treatments (heart failure medications, insulin for type 1 diabetes, steroids for brain swelling, antibiotics, artificial fluids, and nutrition).

- Palliative sedation is a critical last resort option for responding to otherwise very difficult to treat end-of-life suffering. In proportionate palliative sedation, clinicians use the minimal amount of sedation needed to relieve the suffering. A more extreme version, palliative sedation to unconsciousness, is generally reserved for major end-of-life catastrophes (e.g., bleeding out externally and acute agitated delirium at the end of life).
- Voluntarily stopping eating and drinking is an option for those who are still capable of eating and drinking but choose to hasten death by completely stopping both nutrition and hydration.

Who can I consult for professional help?

- In the United States, the American Clinicians Academy on Medical Aid in Dying is a professional society that offers this support.
- Doc2Doc is a professional resource provided by the U.S.-based advocacy organization Compassion & Choices.

CASE RESOLUTION

You have a long discussion with Mrs. Milton at the patient's bedside. He is aphasic and hemiplegic, but he is alert, responds by moving his left arm, and clearly has decisional capacity. It is evident that disease-associated pain, protracted suffering, functional and cognitive decline, loss of dignity and autonomy, inability to engage in enjoyable activities, and fear of burdening his wife underlie his request for PAD. You review his advance directives with his wife, who is his designated health care agent. Dr. Milton has indicated that in the event of a catastrophic illness, he does not wish for futile life-sustaining interventions that will prolong his suffering. He wants to die at home, with only his wife present at his bedside. All his designated financial assets and his body are to be donated to scientific research.

You explain your religious and moral opposition to PAD and discuss other ways to alleviate his suffering. While awaiting a palliative care consult and ethics board review, you intensify his pain and symptom management. Unfortunately, the patient develops intractable seizures, necessitating transfer to inpatient hospice, where his condition progressively declines. With the unanimous agreement of the palliative care team, ethics committee, and his wife, you arrange for him to return home to initiate palliative sedation. A month after he made his request, Dr. Milton is started on a midazolam infusion, titrated gradually to achieve deep sedation and loss of consciousness. Forty-eight hours later, he dies peacefully in his wife's arms, with his favorite Beethoven's *Moonlight Sonata* playing in the background.

Further Reading

1. Abrahm JL. Patient and family requests for hastened death. *Hematology.* 2008;2008(1):475–480. https://doi.org/10.1182/asheducation-2008.1.475
2. American Clinicians Academy on Medical Aid in Dying. Home page. Accessed January 6, 2023. https://www.acamaid.org
3. Compassion & Choices. Doc2Doc. n.d. Accessed January 6, 2023. https://compassionandchoices.org/d2d
4. Death with Dignity. Celebrating a win, creating the future we want: Our 2021 annual report. September 23, 2021. https://deathwithdignity.org/news/2021/09/2021-annual-report
5. University of Missouri School of Medicine. Euthanasia. n.d. Accessed January 5, 2023. https://medicine.missouri.edu/centers-institutes-labs/health-ethics/faq/euthanasia

6. Groenewoud JH, van der Heide A, Onwuteaka-Philipsen BD, Willems DL, van der Maas PJ, van der Wal G. Clinical problems with the performance of euthanasia and physician-assisted suicide in the Netherlands. *N Engl J Med.* 2000;342(8):551–556. doi:10.1056/NEJM200002243420805

7. Lancet Respiratory Medicine. Prolonging life at all costs: Quantity versus quality. *Lancet Respir Medi.* 2016;4(3):165. https://doi.org/10.1016/S2213-2600(16)00059-X

8. Mroz S, Dierickx S, Deliens L, Cohen J, Chambaere K. Assisted dying around the world: A status quaestionis. *Ann Palliat Med.* 2021;10(3):3540553. https://doi.org/10.21037/apm-20-637

9. American Academy of Hospice and Palliative Medicine. Statement on physician-assisted dying. 2016. Accessed December 11, 2022. https://aahpm.org/positions/pad

10. American Medical Association. Physician-assisted suicide. n.d. Accessed December 11, 2022. https://code-medical-ethics.ama-assn.org/ethics-opinions/physician-assisted-suicide

11. Quill TE, Brody RV. "You promised me I wouldn't die like this!" A bad death as a medical emergency. *Arch Intern Med.* 1995;155(12):1250–1254.

12. Wiebe E, Shaw J, Green S, Trouton K, Kelly M. Reasons for requesting medical assistance in dying. *Can Fam Physician.* 2018;64(9):674–679.

13. Worthington A, Finlay I, Regnard C. Efficacy and safety of drugs used for "assisted dying." *Br Med Bull.* 2022;142(1):15–22. doi:10.1093/bmb/ldac009

Further Reading

Readers are encouraged to review "Physician-Assisted Dying" (Up-To-Date), which provides a comprehensive review of the most recent guidelines.

Dr. Timothy Quill (University of Rochester) has written and published extensively on PAD, including 125 journal articles and 35 books.

28 Decision-Making Around Dialysis Withdrawal

Mary K. Buss and Tamara Vesel

Harold is a 42-year-old White man who worked as a construction worker. Fourteen weeks ago, while on a job site, he had a crush injury leading to amputation of three fingers on his dominant hand, splenic infarcts, and internal hemorrhage. His course was complicated by respiratory failure from which he has recovered, multiple infections for which he remains on intravenous antibiotics, and severe acute kidney injury. He has a family history of end-stage renal disease with both his mother, who is now deceased, and his sister receiving hemodialysis. Initially, the team was hopeful that dialysis would be short term. Now he has been on dialysis in the hospital for more than 3 months, and he remains in the intensive care unit (ICU) for some hemodynamic instability. His kidneys show no indication of recovery.

One day, Harold shares with the intern his desire to stop dialysis. "I saw my mom get dialysis for years and my sisters gets it now. I don't want to live like that." When the intern mentions this conversation to other members of the ICU team, they express surprise. "We saved his life. Why would he want to quit?"

What do you do now?

INTRODUCTION

This clinical scenario invites several questions: Why is this patient requesting to stop dialysis? Is he suffering from the dialysis itself? What will happen if he stops dialysis? Will he die? Does he realize that? What is driving the team's reaction to this request? In talking to the renal team, you learn that the patient's life is dependent on dialysis. If dialysis is stopped, he is expected to die within days to a week. In asking these questions, you notice strong reactions from many clinicians on the team. "Dialysis is keeping him alive. If he stops it, he would be committing suicide."

DETERMINING DECISION-MAKING CAPACITY

Whenever a patient voices a preference, especially one that has profound consequences, the health care team has a duty to assess the patient's capacity or competence to make a life-altering decision. At its simplest, capacity requires that the patient understands the consequence of their choice and can provide a rationale for the choice. In this situation, the choice to stop dialysis could lead to death. When a patient expresses a preference that shortens life, it is important to assess whether such a choice is consistent with previously expressed wishes and whether the patient's psychological state is affecting the decision. Finally, any physician can determine if a patient has decision-making capacity for a particular choice. A psychiatrist is not necessary to determine capacity.[1]

When asked why he wants to stop dialysis, Harold expresses frustration with being kept alive just to be on a hospital bed. Although he is grateful to the medical team for all their efforts, he believes that his life is forever changed, and he cannot imagine living life being kept alive on a machine. "I don't want to be kept alive, just to live in the hospital or be on a machine for hours every other day of my life." In assessing Harold's capacity to make this decision, he demonstrates that he understands the consequences of choice. He knows that stopping dialysis will lead to his death. He understands that continuing dialysis will keep him alive. In terms of his rationale, he describes the quality of life on dialysis as unacceptable. He shares the experience of watching his mother on dialysis and feeling that his mother's life was diminished. Harold cannot imagine living that way. He was initially hopeful that dialysis might be temporary, but recently he learned that his kidneys are not expected to recover.

In summary, Harold seems to understand the consequences of a decision not to do dialysis and is able to provide a rationale for his choice. In addition, he is determined not to be depressed, and his views are consistent with values expressed prior to his illness. Thus, Harold has capacity to choose to stop dialysis.

ASSESSING DELIRIUM

Delirium, an alteration in attention that can affect level of consciousness, is highly prevalent in the ICU and often undetected.[2] Diagnosing delirium requires a change in mental status and an inability to maintain attention. There are several validated tools to detect delirium. One of the most common is the Confusion Assessment Method for the Intensive Care Unit (CAM-ICU).[3] To determine if a patient has delirium, this tool first asks if the patient's mental status differs from their baseline. This can be more challenging for patients with underlying dementia or other cognitive disorders. Patients with delirium often have a waxing and waning in mental status. For example, a patient might be alert in the morning and able to respond appropriately to straightforward questions from a physician or nurse, but later in the day they may be overtly confused. Family members may notice more subtle changes missed by the medical team. Patients with more overt delirium may be distracted, answering questions in a tangential fashion or dozing off halfway through a sentence. The most reliable way to assess attention is to conduct a simple test, such as asking a patient to names the days of the week backwards or, for patients on a ventilator, to squeeze your hand each time you say the letter "A" in a string of 10 letters, in which 4 of them are "A"s (e.g., C-A-S-A-B-L-A-N-C-A). Patients who have a change in mental status and fail a test of attention warrant further testing to diagnose delirium. An alteration in either level of consciousness or cognition will make a diagnosis of delirium. Anything other than a normal level of consciousness, ranging from hyperalert to requiring verbal or tactile stimuli to maintain alertness, will confirm delirium. Tests of cognition are only required in patients with a normal level of consciousness and who meet the first two criteria for delirium. Simple yes/no questions such as "Does 1 pound weigh more than 2 pounds?" assess whether a patient is able to think clearly.

Delirium is often categorized as hypoactive or hyperactive. Manifestations of hyperactive delirium include tangential speech, such an incorporating an idea from a nearby conversation into their speech. Such patients often pick at their clothes or pull at foreign objects, such as urinary catheters and intravenous lines. If physically strong enough, they may repeatedly attempt to get out of bed. In contrast, patients with hypoactive delirium are quiet and psychomotor retarded. They may be mistaken for having depression rather than delirium.[2] Some patients vacillate between hypoactive and hyperactive behaviors. Among palliative care patients, hypoactive is more common and likely easier to overlook, making a standardized approach to delirium important to improve detection.

The type of delirium may also affect its management. Despite its prevalence, there are no U.S. Food and Drug Administration–approved medications for delirium. Nonpharmacologic approaches, such as reinforcing typical day and night activities by keeping curtains open during the day and minimizing nighttime disruptions, may prevent delirium among hospitalized patients. Counseling family about common manifestations of delirium and coaching them to offer reassurance to the patient and gently reorientation without directly contradicting the patient are recommended. When patients display dangerous behaviors, such as climbing out of bed, medications may be used to calm them to keep them safe. It is important to recognize that medications are mitigating the agitated behaviors, not treating the delirium. Common medications, including antipsychotics such as haloperidol, olanzapine, or risperidone, should be administered in low doses for as short a period of time as possible. Other medications, such as dexmedetomidine and benzodiazepines, are reserved for patients in whom behaviors persist despite nonpharmacologic and first-line medications.

Returning to our patient, Harold demonstrated delirium early in the course of his ICU stay, but his behavior has since stabilized. He is no longer in restraints, and nursing has not given him any PRN doses of antipsychotics for several weeks. He is attentive on morning rounds and answers questions appropriately. Although this is reassuring, you opt to perform the CAM-ICU, knowing that even patients who are fully oriented can have delirium. On your assessment, he does not meet criteria for delirium. Thus, you have determined that Harold does not have delirium and he does have decision-making capacity. Therefore, he has capacity to decide to stop dialysis. You elect to engage him in a deeper discussion to understand his request to stop dialysis.

GOALS OF CARE

In the context of serious illness, medical decisions can have broad-ranging consequences for both quantity and quality of life. For patients to make truly informed choices about complex medical treatments, they deserve education about the anticipated short-term and long-term consequences as well as the potential risks involved. These conversations are commonly referred to as "goals of care" discussions. They include three key elements: 1) exploring illness understanding, (2) eliciting the patient's goals and values, and (3) making a recommendation based on the first two components.

Exploring Illness Understanding

Although this is primarily aimed at patient understanding, it also requires clarifying the prognosis and anticipated outcomes from all the key members of the medical team. For patients, such as Harold in the ICU, this involves speaking to the various specialists to learn expected outcomes or best- and worst-case scenarios in terms of recovery with respect to organ function, but also overall function. When you speak to the nephrologist for Harold, you learn that despite initial optimism that dialysis would be temporary, he has not had any evidence of kidney recovery and makes no urine on his own. Without dialysis, he is expected to die within 7–10 days. With dialysis, his life would be significantly prolonged, but he would require thrice-weekly hemodialysis. However, the ICU team has struggled to dialyze him due to blood pressure instability and intolerance of hemodialysis. He feels unwell during dialysis sessions, which often last hours. There has been a concerted effort to adjust various aspects of the process and to premedicate him to improve the experience of dialysis without improvement. Due to his chronic osteomyelitis and overall level of illness, he is not currently a candidate for a kidney transplant, and the team is uncertain he would ever meet criteria to be listed for transplant. All specialties agree that he will require additional, extended ICU stay before being transferred to the floor and an extended rehabilitation stay before being able to return home. During this time, he would be at risk for complications that would mean additional time in the hospital.

In talking to Harold, he has a clear understanding that he will die within days to a week or two without dialysis. He describes the dialysis sessions as "torture" and repeatedly has told nurses that he would rather die than continue such sessions three times a week for the rest of his life. He is easily overwhelmed by needles and other medical procedures and has been since early childhood, so peritoneal dialysis does not seem to be an alternative for him. Harold has been evaluated by psychiatry during his hospitalization and deemed not to meet criteria for depression or anxiety disorder.

Eliciting Goals and Values

Before this hospitalization, Harold worked full-time in construction, coached a local sports team, and enjoyed hiking in all seasons. He derived great joy from being active and in nature. Family members recall him making comments about how he could not imagine living without being able to work out. Although saddened, they are not surprised by his request to stop dialysis, stating that they are impressed he has managed this long in the hospital. "This is not how Harold would want to live." Harold has developed a close relationship with the chaplain in the ICU and an intern. He has shared many of his values and sense of his life purpose with each of them.

Making a Recommendation

After clarifying the illness trajectory and eliciting Harold's illness understanding, which is accurate, and exploring Harold's goals and values, you can appreciate why he has made a request to stop dialysis. You talk to him specifically about the limited prognosis once dialysis is stopped and find Harold very ready to talk about the dying process. He has already started the process of saying goodbye to close friends and family members. He asks specific questions about what dying from kidney failure will be like. Before making a recommendation to stop dialysis, you decide to meet with the team.

CARING FOR THE CAREGIVERS

Although caring for patients at the end of life also involves caring for their families, palliative care providers frequently find themselves caring for their colleagues as well. In this clinical scenario, the staff is having more difficulty with Harold's decision than his family. When you meet with some of the ICU team members, they share how "touch and go" Harold's situation was when he first arrived. They prepared the family for his death. At the same time, they continued all aggressive interventions and he "stabilized." During the past 3 weeks, many of his issues have improved. He is no longer delirious and is more alert. They have been able to wean some of his pressors. They have just started to think about transfer to the floor. After weeks in the ICU, they have grown fond of Harold's humor. Several of them express strong feelings of moral obligation for him to continue dialysis in light of everything else that he survived. The nephrology fellow, in particular, cannot understand Harold's decision to forego dialysis—when he might live many years with it. With help from the chaplain who has gotten to know Harold very well, some of the team members acknowledge that his life going forward would be dramatically different than the one he lived before. They start to see all the ways that dialysis will limit him from living the way he values. Although some team members still disagree with the choice, most of them start to understand how it might make sense for Harold, given who he is and how he wants to live. One team member asks, given recent improvements in his care, about delaying the decision for a while.

After meeting with the team, you and a few team members meet with Harold, including the nephrologist, who continues to advocate for dialysis. Harold agrees to another week of aggressive treatment before making a final decision. One week later, Harold remains in the ICU. Although he is "stable overall" by ICU standards, he is not improving, and he has not made it to the floor. He continues to struggle during dialysis. After the agreed time is over, he again requests to stop the dialysis, and his choice is honored.

WITHDRAWAL OF DIALYSIS

Withdrawal of dialysis accounts for 20–25% of deaths among patients on dialysis. Factors associated with requests to cease dialysis include non-Hispanic White race, older age, and comorbid illnesses.[4] The acceptability of withdrawal of dialysis, which was once considered to be suicide, continues to evolve. Nephrologists acknowledge several factors that favor offering or continuing dialysis and do not encourage adequate consideration for patient experience in decisions about dialysis withdrawal.[5] Among patients dependent on dialysis, survival is 7–10 days after withdrawal, leaving limited time for patients to say goodbye to family members, especially because some patients will not be able to communicate due to symptoms of uremic encephalopathy. Although ethically, withdrawal of dialysis or other life-sustaining treatments does not differ from the choice to not initiate such treatment, decisions to withdraw treatment, especially treatments that have succeeded in extending life, can be emotionally challenging for many bedside clinicians.

Anticipating and Managing Symptoms

Pain

Although renal failure does not directly cause pain, patients may have pain from other sources. Acetaminophen is the drug of choice for mild pain. No dose adjustments are needed. With gabapentin, pregabalin, and hydromorphone, toxic metabolites build up when dialysis is stopped, so these agents should be stopped. If opioids are required, methadone and fentanyl are safest. Outside of the hospital, fentanyl may be difficult to administer because it is not absorbed orally. Transdermal patches can be continued. Intravenous or subcutaneous fentanyl can be used for rapid titration and methadone for oral use.

Dyspnea

Dyspnea typically occurs due to accumulation of fluid in the lungs as well as peripherally. Consider diuretics for patients making more than 100 ml of urine daily. A fan in the room or, if hypoxic, supplemental oxygen may help. Otherwise, opioids should be used to palliate dyspnea, which may respond to lower doses than required for pain (see the section titled "Pain").

Nausea

Metoclopramide effectively treats nausea, which may result from underlying gastroparesis. Ondansetron is also commonly used and may be less sedating than other antiemetics. Patients may be more susceptible to nausea from other medications, such as opioids, so antiemetics should be used pro-actively prior to dosing opioids.[6]

Encephalopathy

Sedation and confusion are expected as the toxins, cleared by the kidney, build up. Unless the patient exhibits behaviors that are unsafe or upsetting to family members (see the section titled "Assessing Delirium"), the best approach is to create a calm environment and educate family about the ex-pected changes.

Agitation, Anxiety, and Restlessness

Agitation and restlessness are outward manifestations of encephalopathy and anxiety that a patient may no longer be able to verbalize. If behaviors are unsafe, leading to the risk of falls, or disturbing to family members, medications can be initiated. Dose adjustments may be needed. For ex-ample, haloperidol dose should be halved. Because the goal is comfort, more sedating antipsychotics such as olanzapine or quetiapine may be pre-ferred. Benzodiazepines do not require dose adjustments.[6]

Adjusting Other Medications

Any medications not actively contributing to comfort should be dis-continued. This includes most, if not all, medications other than ones addressing the symptoms mentioned previously, and it limits the need to administer pills by mouth, as the patient is expected to lose the ability to swallow as the end approaches.

Preparing the Family

Loved ones generally want to know what to expect regarding the time frame and the patient experience. Most family members are relieved to learn that patients rarely develop pain and often have limited symptoms, just a fading away. Helping families anticipate the potential for changes in mental status, which can manifest as confusion, as well as alteration in personality in early stages is important so that family members can help calm and redirect the patient. In addition, it is important for family members to know that the period of lucidity may be shorter than the life expectancy. Loved ones are encouraged to communicate love and gratitude and also to offer and request forgiveness. For some, saying goodbye might include giving the patient permission to die and/or offering reassurance that the family member will be okay after the death. If the patient is dying at home, family members may require more education about anticipation and management of symptoms, administration of medications, and provision of custodial care.

CASE RESOLUTION

Knowing his time was short, Harold wanted to focus on time with his family. The ICU team was able to simplify his care to focus on comfort. He was transferred to a nearby inpatient hospice house, where he died a few days later with his family present.

KEY POINTS TO REMEMBER

- Decision-making capacity requires that the patient understands the consequence of their choice and can provide a rationale for the choice.
- Delirium, an alteration in attention that can but does not always affect level of consciousness, is prevalent and often undetected among patients in the ICU.
- For patients to make truly informed choices about complex medical treatments, clinicians should engage patients in "goals of care" discussions that include (1) exploring illness understanding, (2) eliciting the patient's goals and values, and (3) making a recommendation based on the first two components.
- Withdrawal of dialysis accounts for nearly 25% of deaths among patients on dialysis. Among patients dependent on dialysis, average survival is 7–10 days after withdrawal.
- Common symptoms in patients dying from renal failure include encephalopathy, dyspnea and edema from fluid overload, pain, nausea, and agitation or restlessness. Medications, dose-adjusted for renal dysfunction, can successfully mitigate these symptoms.

References

1. Ehrman SE, Norton KP, Karol DE, et al. Top ten tips palliative care clinicians should know about medical decision-making capacity assessment. *J Palliat Med.* 2021;24(4):599–604.

2. Stollings J, Kotfis K, Chanques G, Pun BT, Pandharipande PP, Ely EE. Delirium in critical illness: Clinical manifestations, outcomes, and management. *Intensive Care Med.* 2021;47(10):1089–1103.

3. Chanques G, Ely EW, Garnier O, et al. The 2014 updated version of the Confusion Assessment Method for the Intensive Care Unit compared to the 5th version of the Diagnostic and Statistical Manual of Mental Disorders and other current methods used by intensivists. *Ann Intensive Care.* 2018;8(1):33.

4. Agunbiade A, Dasgupta A, Ward M. Racial/ethnic differences in dialysis discontinuation and survival after hospitalization for serious conditions among patients on maintenance dialysis. *J Am Soc Nephrol.* 2020;31:149–160.

5. Grubbs V, Tuot DS, Powe NR, O'Donoghue D, Chesla CA. System-level barriers and facilitators for foregoing or withdrawing dialysis: A qualitative study of nephrologists in the United States and England. *Am J Kidney Dis.* 2017;70(5):602–610.

6. Davison SN, Rosielle DA. Fast Fact #208: Clinical care following withdrawal of dialysis. Palliative Care Network of Wisconsin. October 2008. Accessed January 19, 2023. https://www.mypcnow.org/fast-fact/clinical-care-following-withdrawal-of-dialysis

Further Reading

Gelfand SL, Scherer JS, Koncicki HM. Kidney supportive care: Core curriculum 2020. *Am J Kidney Dis.* 2020;75(5):793–806.

29 LGBTQ: To Disclose or Not to Disclose

Gabriel Lutz

Mark is being evaluated on the general medicine inpatient service for new onset of significant fatigue, night sweats, unintentional weight loss, and new oral thrush. Further evaluation demonstrates positive HIV serum titers and a large intracranial mass that biopsy demonstrates to be central nervous system lymphoma not amenable to traditional therapy. Mark is distraught over the news of his diagnosis, as is his family, which consists of both parents. His family would like to discuss the possibility of enrolling in an experimental, high-risk clinical trial. You recommend a family meeting with the oncology consultant and Mark's family to discuss his prognosis and treatment options.

Mark is a single, gay man. He previously named his parents as his health care agents for medical decision-making. He confides in you that his family knows about his lymphoma but not about his HIV diagnosis nor about his sexual orientation. He explains that his family is hostile toward the LGBTQ community, and he worries that revealing his HIV status will inevitably lead to a discussion about his sexual orientation. Mark states he would rather die than come out as gay to his family.

What do you do now?

DISCUSSION

Among the founding principles of modern bioethics, the principle of respecting an individual patient's autonomy is of great importance. Respect for autonomy entails respecting the choices an individual makes for themself, granted they are without cognitive impairment, without coercion, and they are informed of the likely outcomes.[1] The ethical principle of autonomy gives rise to the subsequent principle of confidentiality, which holds that physicians are obligated not to share a patient's health information unless given explicit permission from the patient.[1] Confidentiality is also a core component of the American Medical Association's code of ethics.[2]

Although each is significant in their own right, none of the primary ethical principles (autonomy, justice, beneficence, and nonmaleficence) is of superior importance in relation to the others—they must be practiced in balance with each other.[3] Ethical dilemmas occur when these principles come into conflict, requiring a nuanced evaluation of the contextual details of a given patient case. For example, the right to confidentiality can be overridden if sharing private health knowledge would confer a benefit to general society that outweighs the benefit of individual privacy.[1] Although several health conditions are required to be reported by the Centers for Disease Control and Prevention, including certain infectious diseases such as new HIV diagnoses, these notifiable reports are not personally identifiable and therefore do not violate confidentiality.[4] Threats to an individual's confidentiality, and by extension to their autonomy, occur when private health information is shared unknowingly or in contradiction to their request for privacy.

In this scenario, respecting Mark's wish for confidentiality will not cause harm to anyone in his family, but violation is likely to cause great emotional harm to Mark. Specifically, violation of Mark's confidentiality will erode his sense of safety and support from his family, greatly decreasing his quality of life and potential for recovery. When faced with a difficult decision, it is always wise to consider the overall harms and benefits to each party involved and to proceed with the solution that honors the four founding ethical principles and results in the greatest benefit and least harm.

CASE RESOLUTION

Given that Mark is an adult with decision-making capacity requesting specific privacy, all attempts at honoring this request should be made. His decision to focus first on the more urgent threat of metastatic malignancy, while addressing a less urgent infection privately, is understandable. Although no readily available cure for HIV infection currently exists, it has become a manageable chronic condition through the use of highly efficacious antiretroviral medications. Therefore, the upcoming family meeting should remain focused on exploring Mark's cancer treatment options and overall goals. In this way, trust and empathic relationship-building will greatly aid Mark in navigating his personal health journey. It may also empower Mark to build enough confidence to foster open communication and potentially come out to his family in the future.

KEY POINTS TO REMEMBER

- Patient autonomy is a foundational ethical principle that all providers should respect.
- The duty to respect patient confidentiality is explicitly required by law unless other compelling legal circumstances exist (risk of child/adult harm or neglect, risk of violence to others, and risk of communicable infectious disease spread).
- Providers should sensitively assess a patient's needs, both medical and emotional. When possible, peaceful shared decision-making should be the goal of family meetings.

References
1. Macauley RC. *Ethics in Palliative Care*. Oxford University Press; 2018:34–39.
2. American Medical Association. Patient's rights. n.d. Accessed January 3, 2023. https://code-medical-ethics.ama-assn.org/ethics-opinions/patient-rights
3. Beauchamp TL, Childress JF. Respect for autonomy. In: *Principles of Biomedical Ethics*. 8th ed. Oxford University Press; 2019:99–154.
4. Centers for Disease Control and Prevention. Notifiable infectious disease tables. October 24, 2022. Accessed December 19, 2023. https://www.cdc.gov/nndss/data-statistics/infectious-tables

30 Can Minors Make Major Medical Decisions?

Sudha Chandrasekhar

Diya Shankar is a 15-year-old high school sophomore. You have been her trusted primary care pediatrician since her birth. Academically excelling, captain of her school swim team, a gifted violinist, and Indian classical dancer, Diya is debating pursuing a professional career in science versus art. She was diagnosed with osteogenic sarcoma of the right proximal humerus at age 13½ years, which initially responded to a brutal treatment regimen of limb-sparing surgery, radiation, and chemotherapy while only briefly impacting her academic and extracurricular activities. Eight months later, her tumor recurred and spread into her shoulder joint and right lung. The oncologist recommends amputation of the right arm above the shoulder joint, followed by more aggressive chemotherapy and immunotherapy, and eventually to be fitted with a prosthetic device. When Diya hears the side effects of the treatment and the slim chance of success, she asks you, "I'm going to die from this cancer, right? I'll never be able to play the violin or perform my dance debut. I don't want this treatment. I just want to enjoy my life, not go through that hell again." Her parents argue, plead, and fight with her in vain to consent to the treatment. They beg you to persuade her to continue fighting for her life. But Diya angrily refuses and asks you. "It's my body. It's my life. Why can't it be my choice?"

What do you do now?

DISCUSSION

The adolescent years, from ages 10 to 19 years, mark the transition from childhood to adulthood. Adolescence encompasses an array of cognitive, physical, sexual, and developmental milestones that are unique to this age group. It is the age of emerging autonomy when adolescents begin to separate from their parents, find their own identity, and think independently. Autonomy is the ability to feel, behave, and think independently. Autonomy is a sense of self-governance or freedom to make choices. Adolescents raised in an environment that fosters these critical developmental milestones can engage in collaborative communication and facilitated decision-making. Providing age-appropriate anticipatory guidance that helps parents and adolescents develop such skills is the responsibility of all clinicians who care for children.

Among adolescents, those with childhood cancer form a distinct subsect. Cancer is the fourth leading cause of death in this age group, behind accidents, suicide, and homicide. The American Cancer Society estimates that approximately 500–600 adolescents die from cancer each year. Osteosarcoma (OS) accounts for approximately 3% of all cancers in teens aged 15–19 years. Approximately 800 new cases of OS are reported each year in the United States, half of which are in children and teens. Treatment options for OS include limb-sparing surgery, chemotherapy, radiation, and targeted therapy when detected in the early stages. Recurrent OS often necessitates radical surgery, including amputation of the affected limb.

The overall 5-year survival rate for children ages 0–19 years with OS is 68%. The stage of the tumor at the time of diagnosis, local versus distant spread, and the unique tumor pathology, as well as individual response to treatment, determine 5-year survival. Metastatic OS has a 5-year survival rate of 27%. Recurrent cancer within 18 months is more refractory to treatment and drops the survival rate to 17%.

The lived experiences of childhood cancer create a subsect of adolescents who are biologically and psychologically distinct both from their healthy peers and from adults with cancer. Accelerated cognitive maturation in seriously ill children often allows adequate capacity and judgment to engage effectively in the informed consent or refusal process for proposed goals of care; grasp the realities of their illness; understand the risks, consequences, and nature of treatment; and acknowledge the meaning and finality of death.

Traditionally, parents are vested with legal authority as unilateral decision-makers for children younger than age 18 years. Parents are believed to act in the child's best interests. But emerging neuroscientific research on developing brain structures in minors shows that by age 12 years, children have acquired the four critical capacities required for decision-making, namely communicating a choice, understanding, reasoning, and appreciation. Such capacity forms the basis of the "mature minor doctrine," the common-law rule that allows an adolescent who is mature to give consent for medical care. Critical elements of the mature minor doctrine include age older than 14 years and demonstrated capacity for informed decision-making.

Yet, this age coincides with emerging adolescence, in which early development of the brain's reward system, combined with later development of the control system, may diminish decision-making competence in specific contexts. Thus, although adolescents may possess decision-making ability, they still need the support of parents, caregivers, and clinicians to facilitate these emerging skills.

Clinicians caring for children should help families understand that parental authority is not absolute. Rather, it should be constrained by respect of the child. Lainie Friedman Ross' model of constrained parental autonomy describes parents as surrogate decision-makers who balance the best interest of the minor patient with the family's best interests, as long as the child's basic medical needs are met. Moving the conversation from parental rights toward parental responsibility promotes collaborative communication. It provides a framework for clinicians to help families minimize conflicts encountered in the course of more serious and difficult medical decision-making.

Medical decision-making is not a discrete event. It evolves over time among the health care team, family, and pediatric patient as new information becomes available. Pediatric practice is unique in that developmental maturation allows, over time, for increasing inclusion of the child's and adolescent's opinion in medical decision-making. Thus, shared family-centered decision-making is increasingly recommended in pediatric decision-making. It is an invaluable tool for children and families facing serious, unexpected, life-limiting illness.

Myra Bluebond-Langer's work offers valuable insights when families and clinicians have to face a child's unexpected life-threatening, life-shortening illness. In parents, overwhelming disbelief slowly turns to fear, grief, and despair. Their natural instincts as nurturers, fierce advocates, and protectors come to the forefront. They channel their energies into leaving no stone unturned. Parents may realize when cure is not possible. But they willingly choose options with infinitesimal odds because the prize they seek—their child's life—has immeasurable value to them. Just as a child's identity is shaped by serious illness, so also parents forge their identity through this challenging experience. Illness becomes the context that defines what it means to be a parent.

Physicians also experience deep sorrow when children they care for are diagnosed with life-altering illnesses. Profound grief stems from their role as professional and personal partners with the child and family, through years of nurturing and caregiving. While physicians who are themselves parents can express great empathy, they may also experience intense fear about their own children being similarly affected. Involving children in difficult treatment and decisional conversations may demand clinicians asking them to make a "choiceless choice," requiring them to say and hear things that are excruciatingly painful. Yet, challenging as it may be, there is implicit value in talking to and listening to a child, without focusing on a particular outcome.

An emotionally charged dilemma arises when an adolescent refuses a treatment or intervention that is advocated by the parent(s) and often the treating clinician(s). The shuttle diplomacy model proposed by Bluebond-Langner et al. provides a valuable framework that strives to ensure that all participants are represented and can negotiate mutually acceptable trade-offs, leading to satisfactory conflict resolution.

The American Academy of Pediatrics (AAP) Committee on Bioethics' "Informed Consent in Decision-Making in Pediatric Practice"[11] is a landmark policy statement. It provides a framework for informed consent, permission, and assent in pediatrics, akin to Bluebond-Langner's shuttle diplomacy approach (Box 30.1).

Key Recommendations of the AAP Policy Statement

Physicians should involve pediatric patients in their health care decision-making by providing information on their illness and options for diagnosis and treatment in a developmentally appropriate manner and seeking assent to medical care whenever appropriate.

Parents should generally be recognized as the appropriate ethical and legal surrogate medical decision-makers for their children and adolescents. This recognition affirms parents' intimate understanding of their children's interests and respects the importance of family autonomy.

Surrogate decision-making by parents or guardians for pediatric patients should seek to maximize benefits for the child by balancing health care needs with social and emotional needs within the context of overall family goals, religious and cultural beliefs, and values.

Physicians should recognize that some pediatric patients, especially older adolescents and those with medical experience from chronic illness, may possess adequate capacity, cognitive ability, and judgment to engage effectively in the informed consent or refusal process for proposed goals of care.

The dilemma of an adolescent treatment refusal is ethically and emotionally challenging. Instances in which treatment burdens may outweigh benefits and fail to achieve a curative end should mandate thoughtful guidance from the physician, with continued communication among the patient, surrogates, and health care team to clarify values and treatment goals. Knowledge of individual state laws on adolescent treatment refusals is critical in these situations.

Physicians have both a moral obligation and a legal responsibility to question and, if necessary, to contest both the surrogate's and the patient's medical decisions if they put the patient at significant risk of serious harm.

Physicians must realize that informed consent/permission/assent/refusal constitutes a process, not a discrete event, and requires the sharing of information in ongoing physician–patient–family communication and education.

Physicians must have access to and understanding of their specific state statutes governing the definition and care of the emancipated minor and adolescents who possess decision-making capacity (mature minors), with critical attention to adolescent confidentiality.

Reproduced from the AAP.[11]

CASE RESOLUTION

You arrange a meeting with Diya's oncologist, pediatric surgeon, and Diya's parents. Divya's parents are shocked, refusing to accept that Diya's cancer has recurred. They are angry that the first round of treatment was not aggressive enough. Diya's mother recoils in horror about her child's body being mutilated, but Diya's father gently reminds her that it is a small price to pay for Diya's life. Her parents insist that it is not culturally acceptable for the health care team to discuss treatment options with her alone, irately stating, "We have no secrets in our family."

Your team meets with Diya in her room. You are seated on her bed holding her hand as you speak, while her parents are hovering anxiously at the foot of her bed. Diya listens quietly, turns toward you, and buries her face in her pillow. In a muffled voice, she declares,

> I hate cancer. I hate my life. I know I'm going to die. I don't want to look like a freak with my arm cut off. It's my body. It's my life. And it's my choice. I just don't care anymore.

Diya's parents plead with her to reconsider. After much discussion, Diya tearfully agrees to go through chemotherapy and radiation but not the limb amputation. The oncologist explains that the amputation may be the only possible way to save her life. Diya answers, "I don't want to live looking like a mutilated one-arm freak."

Diya starts the next grueling round of chemotherapy, radiation, and immunotherapy. She writes about her experiences daily in an online blog and pours her emotions into words. Six weeks into the treatment, Diya develops septic shock and cardiac arrest from which she cannot be resuscitated. At her funeral, Diya's parents give you a letter she wrote you the day before she died. It reads, "Dear Dr. Gupta: Thank you for listening to me and hearing my voice. I will never forget you. Love Diya."

KEY POINTS TO REMEMBER

· Informed consent is an essential component of health care practice.

- Seeking parental permission and adolescent consent is an active family-centric process.
- Medical decision-making is neither a static nor discrete event. It evolves over time among the health care team, family, and pediatric patient as new information becomes available.
- Pediatric practice is unique because it takes into account the developmental maturation of the child in the context of unexpected life-altering illness.
- Including the adolescent promotes shared decision-making, facilitates teamwork, and has the potential to dimmish family conflicts.
- Clinicians who care for children have a moral and ethical responsibility to advocate for each child in a manner that is commensurate with their development.
- Clinicians can experience profound distress when their patient is unexpectedly diagnosed with a serious, potentially life-limiting illness. In order to heal and move forward effectively, clinicians must look into self-care options that allow for introspection, debriefing, and healing.

References

1. Alderman EM, Breuner CC, Committee on Adolescence. Unique needs of the adolescent. *Pediatrics*. 2019;144(6):e20193150. https://doi.org/10.1542/peds.2019-3150
2. Bluebond-Langner M, Belasco JB, Goldman A, Belasco C. Understanding parents' approaches to care and treatment of children with cancer when standard therapy has failed. *J Clin Oncol*. 2007;25(17):2414–2419. doi:10.1200/JCO.2006.08.7759
3. Dattilo TM, Olshefski RS, Nahata L, Hansen-Moore JA, Gerhardt CA, Lehmann V. Growing up after childhood cancer: Maturity and life satisfaction in young adulthood. *Support Care Cancer*. 2021;29(11):6661–6668. doi:10.1007/s00520-021-06260-3
4. Day E, Jones L, Langner R, Bluebond-Langner M. Current understanding of decision-making in adolescents with cancer: A narrative systematic review. *Palliat Med*. 2016;30(10):920–934. https://doi.org/10.1177/0269216316648072
5. Grootens-Wiegers P, Hein IM, van den Broek JM, de Vries MC. Medical decision-making in children and adolescents: Developmental and neuroscientific aspects. *BMC Pediatr*. 2017;17:120. https://doi.org/10.1186/s12887-017-0869-x

6. Katz S. A minor's right to die with dignity: The ultimate act of love, compassion, mercy, and civil liberty. *Calif West Int Law J*. 2018;48(2):3.

7. King NM, Cross AW. Children as decision makers: Guidelines for pediatricians. *J Pediatr*. 1989;115(1):10–16. doi:10.1016/s0022-3476(89)80321-x

8. Mack JW, Joffe S, Hilden JM, et al. Parents' views of cancer-directed therapy for children with no realistic chance for cure. *J Clin Oncol*. 2008;26(29):4759–4764. https://doi.org/10.1200/JCO.2007.15.6059

9. Sigman GS, O'Connor C. Exploration for physicians of the mature minor doctrine. *J Pediatr*. 1991;119(4):520–525. doi:10.1016/s0022-3476(05)82398-4

10. American Cancer Society. Key statistics for cancers in adolescents. n.d. https://www.cancer.org/cancer/types/cancer-in-children/key-statistics.html

11. American Academy of Pediatrics, Committee on Bioethics. Informed consent in decision-making in pediatric practice. *Pediatrics*. 2016;*138*(2):e20161484. https://publications.aap.org/pediatrics/article/138/2/e20161484/52512/Informed-Consent-in-Decision-Making-in-Pediatric?autologincheck=redirected

Further Reading

Readers are encouraged to refer to the comprehensive AAP policy statement for guidelines regarding informed consent in pediatric medical decision-making. Myra Bluebond-Langer's pioneering work on shuttle diplomacy offers a practical, diplomatic, negotiated approach to shared pediatric medical decision-making.

Surrogate Decision-Making

Margaret M. Mahon

Mr. Allen is an 86-year-old widow who lives alone. His children have not visited in 3 years, but they call. They have realized that their father cannot follow conversations and forgets with whom he is speaking.

Neighbors check on Mr. Allen, and he receives Meals on Wheels. He is fiercely private, not allowing people into his home. When Mr. Allen did not answer his door for 3 days, the police did a wellness check; Mr. Allen was found down. At the hospital, he was diagnosed with an intertrochanteric hip fracture. When surgery to stabilize the fracture is recommended, Mr. Allen yells, "You're not doing anything to me! Let me go home!"

He is combative and believes that people are trying to harm him. Mr. Allen does not recognize his children when they arrive. Police reported that the home was cluttered, with food and dirty laundry throughout. The attending suggests that Mr. Allen has advanced dementia.

His children are reluctant to encourage their father to consent for surgery, nor are they willing to sign the consent for his surgery as long as he declines. One read on the internet that conservative management is appropriate for hip fractures.

The staff are very concerned that Mr. Allen is not undergoing surgery.

What do you do now?

CLINICAL DECISION-MAKING

Mr. Allen's situation is complex. The most important step in clinical decision-making is determining what questions need to be answered and then answering them. Perhaps the fundamental question is whether Mr. Allen is capable of refusing surgery (an informed refusal). Listening to what he has said in the emergency department (ED), it sounds like Mr. Allen is adamant about not undergoing surgical repair. Inarguably, dementia affects decision-making. Clinicians must consider *how* dementia affects informed consent for Mr. Allen. If he cannot consent, who can or should consent (or refuse) for him? Dementia may be more closely scrutinized if it impedes the usual plan of care or if the patient chooses not to follow against providers' recommendations.

DEFINITIONS

Many factors affect the process of medical decision-making. Although not all of these factors are used in every situation, it is important to be able to integrate salient considerations as necessary for each patient's clinical situation. It is also important to identify when certain factors do not apply in a specific situation.

Advance Directives

An *advance directive* is a means to convey health care preferences before they are needed. (Note that they are *advance* directives, because they are done in advance, not *advanced* directives.) Not all advance directives require a lawyer. The presence of a legal document is far less important than understanding the patient's preferences.

Types of advance directives include

- a living will;
- a durable power of attorney for health care;
- a do not attempt resuscitation (DNAR) or do not resuscitate document;
- an informal document, such as a letter written by a patient in which the patient has identified preferences for clinical care and/or a surrogate; and

- statements made to others expressing preferences for care and/or identification of a surrogate.

At its most basic, an advance directive accomplishes two things: naming a surrogate (someone to represent the patient's preferences in decision-making) and identifying the individual's preferences for clinical care. Advance directives are most commonly used when a patient is unable to make decisions, but they can also inform situations in which a patient chooses not to participate in decision-making.[1]

Capacity

Capacity refers to the ability to give informed consent; it is a clinical judgment. Capacity can be assessed by a range of clinicians; a psychiatrist is not required in most cases. An assessment of capacity can be done using the "four C's"[2]:

- **Comprehension:** Can the patient comprehend the condition and the resultant choices?
- **Consideration:** Is the patient able to weigh options? This requires balancing. It requires considering the effects of each choice.
- **Choose:** Is the patient able to make a decision? Is the decision consistent with what is known about the person's history and values? In this case, the first choice is about surgery: whether or not to have it.
- **Consistent communication:** Does the patient express a decision consistently? A patient with capacity will report the same answer to the same question to different people.

Competence

Clinicians, lawyers, family members, and others sometimes use the terms *competence* and *capacity* interchangeably. They are not the same. Whereas capacity is a clinical decision about the patient's ability to participate in decision-making about one's own care, competence is a legal decision. A judge decides whether a person is competent or not, based on evidence provided. Competence is not a global decision; a person might be adjudicated competent to make medical decisions but not competent to make financial decisions.

Informed Consent

Informed consent is a process through which a patient is given the information necessary to make a decision about a health care intervention, and the patient decides. The process requires that an informed person gives the patient enough information to make a decision and that the patient is able and willing to make the decision. Patients must be able to understand the information provided, and the decision must be voluntary.[3]

Informed Refusal

Like informed consent, *informed refusal* is also a process. A person should use the same information that comprises informed consent: does the patient understand the information and voluntarily choose whether to undergo the procedure. Or not.

Surrogate

Surrogate is derived from the Latin *surrogare*, "to put in another's place." Sometimes the definition is written as "to stand in the shoes of." Often in health care, when a patient is not able or chooses not to participate in health care decision-making, a surrogate is brought in to the discussion. Often, however, we say to the parent, sibling, or child of the patient, "What do you want us to do?" This is the wrong question because it focuses the decision on the *family member's* opinion or decision. The role of the surrogate is to represent the *patient's* wishes in decision-making. By asking the question differently, we guide and even allow the family member (or whomever is there *for the patient*) to represent the patient's wishes. It is our responsibility to ask the right question that allows another to function as a surrogate.

Mr. Allen said he does not want surgery. His children clearly want the best for him. To allow them to act as surrogates, we must structure the question to allow them to represent his wishes. Ideally, this will unburden them, allowing them to act *in his stead*, rather than making the decision themselves.[4] "Your father has said he does not want surgery. You know we are concerned that dementia is affecting his thinking right now. Before his thinking changed, what do you think he would have said?" Or, "If we went back 10 years, what do you think your father would have wanted in this situation?" Structuring the questions this way allows, even challenges, those acting *in the shoes of* the patient to focus on the patient's wishes rather than their own.

Substituted Judgment

Substituted judgment is related to the concept of surrogacy. The premise for both is that decision-making is an opportunity to respect the patient's autonomy. (The term *autonomy* derives from the Latin *auto* + *nomos*: self rule. Providers must respect the patient's autonomy. Providers or surrogates are not bound by it but, rather, must acknowledge and respect it.) Those representing the patient in decision-making (in this case, Mr. Allen's children) should make a decision based on what they believe the patient would decide. That is, knowing the patient's values and beliefs, what do the surrogates believe the patient would want?

In Mr. Allen's case, the challenge of substituted judgment is not just to respect Mr. Allen's wishes but also to consider factors that he might not have been able to contemplate. Did Mr. Allen ever imagine that his thinking would be compromised? That he might not live alone safely? How do the children consider his apparent change in preferences over years?

Supported Decision-Making

Supported decision-making is typically undertaken with the expectation that a person's ability to participate in decision-making is or may become compromised. The person (the beneficiary) identifies a person or people (the supporters) who will help in decision-making.[5] The agreement can be formal (a written document that might be shared with health care providers, long-term care administrators, or others) or informal, shared knowledge based on a discussion. Supported decision-making is a way to construct a team of decision-makers. If the patient cannot participate and cannot benefit from the input from the supporters, then supported decision-making is not an option.[3] If the patient cannot participate as a member of the team, the team is disbanded.

APPLICATIONS OF THE PRINCIPLES TO MR. ALLEN'S CASE

Who Decides?

When the patient is unable to participate fully in decision-making, ideally a foundation has been laid by prior discussions about future health care.[6] This allows the surrogates to decide based on previously identified preferences. Mr. Allen is unable to say whether he has any kind of advance directive. His children reported that they know he has a will. When their mother, the patient's wife, died 7 years ago, Mr. Allen's children remember that he said, "Your mother and I took care of everything. We have all the paperwork." Mr. Allen's wife died from cancer; she received hospice care at home for 3 weeks before she died. Decisions requiring an advance directive, surrogacy, or substituted judgment were never necessary.

Based on Mr. Allen's statements, one of Mr. Allen's children called the patient's attorney, Ms. Clarkson. Ms. Clarkson stated that Mr. Allen's will included a durable power of attorney for health care document. Mr. Allen had named his wife as his surrogate decision-maker. Unfortunately, the document was never updated.

Mr. Allen's advance directive identified several preferences in the form of a living will. Specifically, Mr. Allen specified that were he unable to make or communicate decisions, his surrogate could make decisions "to withhold or withdraw medical care and surgical procedures, [including] . . . nutrition or hydration, . . . antibiotics, . . . blood products, . . . artificial respiration." The document applied to end-of-life decisions. This type of advance directive presumes that the surrogate would know what the patient would want were the patient unable to decide. Likely, his wife would have known; however, Mr. Allen never had these discussions with his children.

It is agreed that Mr. Allen cannot given informed consent or informed refusal. Specifically, he cannot retain the information he is given. He cannot weigh the benefits and burdens of any option. Mr. Allen is unable to communicate any understanding. He consistently declines surgery, but his refusals seem reflexive and fear-based. He is also unable to participate in supported decision-making. He is, however, consistent in his refusal of surgery, and he is adamant in his desire to return home.

His three children are present. The ED attending, the patient's nurse, and the orthopedic surgeon have spoken with the children; the health care team agree that the children want what is best for Mr. Allen, that they will act in his best interest, considering what they know of their father and what they hear from the providers. The children agree to "help him decide." All involved agree that the children will be Mr. Allen's surrogates. So, what is next?

Physiologic Data

In clinical decision-making, patient preferences and provider preferences are not the sole considerations; respect for autonomy is not the only principle to be considered. Autonomy exists only in the context of accurate physiologic data. No decision should be made based solely on patient preferences. The foundation for clinical decision-making must include the facts about Mr. Allen's anatomy, physiology, and treatment.

The children need information about Mr. Allen's conditions: his hip fracture in the context of dementia. The ED physician, Dr. Jeffreys, explained the patient's hip fracture and showed them Mr. Allen's X-rays. She reiterated her understanding of the need for surgery. She explained that she had never taken care of a patient with hip fracture who did not have surgery. Dr. Jeffreys said that she believed Mr. Allen would heal better with surgery.

Because the children were still reluctant, the orthopedic surgeon, Dr. Michaels, came to speak with the family. He said that he strongly recommended surgery. He described the surgery, saying that it was routine and fairly simple, involving insertion of an intramedullary hip screw for Mr. Allen's unstable hip fracture. Dr. Michaels explained that although he strongly recommended surgery, it was not without risks. Patients with dementia who fracture a hip and who undergo surgery are at significantly higher risk for complications than people with hip fracture without dementia. This includes increased postoperative risk of respiratory complications, cardiovascular complications, sepsis, and death.[7,8]

Mr. Allen's children are surprised that he will not consent to surgery. "He would do anything that would allow him to be able to live on his own." They understand the recommendation for surgery, however, they also believe that Mr. Allen means what he says: He does not want surgery and he wants to go home. Their struggle is to balance physiologic data and risks with their father's apparent changes in preferences.

Ideally, the process of decision-making starts before illness impedes decision-making abilities. We each should consider what we would want in health care situations (patient preferences), as well as who could represent our wishes were we unable to (or choose not to) express our preferences (identification of a surrogate).[1] Mr. Allen had started the process; he and his wife had advance directives. Because Mr. Allen had not updated his medical power of attorney, the children are in the position of acting as surrogates, doing their best to respect their father's wishes.

It is common for people with dementia to change their preferences for care as the disease progresses. In these cases, clinicians often do not know how to guide family decision-making: whether the patient's preferences before or early in the patient's course of dementia or currently expressed preferences should be given more weight. This is the quandary Mr. Allen's children are facing. While they agree that their father would previously have consented to surgery, his thoughts seem different now.

The first reaction of many health care providers is that surgery is the only viable option for Mr. Allen. Patients and families are often told that surgery is the only option; however, conservative management is a reasonable option.

Because they were still grappling with what was the right thing to do, Dr. Jeffreys consulted a geriatrician, Dr. Roberts. Researchers found that following a consult with a geriatrician for patients older than age 70 years with hip fracture, a decision to *decline* surgical intervention increased from 2.7% to 9.1% (p = .008).[9] Dr. Roberts examined Mr. Allen. She explained to the family that she believes he has had many falls, noting the presence of several bruises and scrapes on his knees, hips, and forearms.

Dr. Roberts is able to expand the context of decision-making. That is, she reminded the children that they were not just making a decision about surgery but also about their father's broader life. Dementia at an advanced stage means that Mr. Allen likely cannot return home safely. So, even if the children wanted to respect Mr. Allen's wishes—"Just let me go home!"—he can no longer live there, or at least not alone.

People with dementia are significantly less likely to be able to walk independently or with assistance following hip fracture. They are also at significantly increased risk for postoperative infection, delirium, joint dislocation, respiratory complications, anesthetic complications, and even death.[8,10,11]

Surgery also is not without complications. Patients with dementia who fracture a hip and who do have surgery are at significantly higher risk for respiratory complications, cardiovascular complications, sepsis, and death.[7,8]

DECIDING FOR MR. ALLEN

Mr. Allen's children were distressed about several issues, especially what they perceived as a marked change in their father's preferences. Mr. Allen, who previously would have done anything to stay home, including surgery, was now adamantly opposed to surgery. Mr. Allen's children accepted that he really did not want surgery.

Their father's advanced dementia was the children's greatest source of distress. They were embarrassed and felt guilty that they were unaware of how much his condition, both cognitive and physical, had declined. They also realized that he could not return home, even if he were to have surgery. It would not be safe.

The children opted for conservative management. Mr. Allen was admitted; his hip was immobilized. After initial immobilization in the hospital, Mr. Allen was transferred to subacute rehabilitation for the duration of his healing. Mr. Allen's children and the staff were surprised that he was calm and comfortable. He especially enjoyed meals and snacks. Dr. Roberts, the geriatrician, discussed code status with the family; a DNAR order was placed.

A palliative care consultation was placed. Mr. Allen's pain was well managed. He had a femoral nerve block and was started on around-the-clock acetaminophen and low-dose oxycodone (2.5 mg p.o. q 4 hr prn). He used approximately one dose per day.

On day 4, Mr. Allen acutely developed shortness of breath and tachypnea. He was less responsive. The nurse placed him on 4 L of oxygen, and workup for pulmonary embolism was started. He was given a single dose of intravenous fentanyl (25 μg) for shortness of breath. In the emergency department, because of his age, dementia, and apparent delirium no benzodiazepines were administered. Mr. Allen was peaceful and comfortable. He died approximately 90 minutes later.

The patient's children are appropriately sad about his death, but they are relieved that "we didn't make him have surgery." He was comfortable and surrounded by family for his last days. He usually did not recognize his children, but he enjoyed having visitors.

- The role of the surrogate is to act "in the shoes" of another person when that person is unable or chooses not to participate in decision-making.
- Health care providers are responsible for asking the right questions. Not, "What do you want us to do?" but, rather, "If your father were able to talk with us right now, if he were thinking as he did prior to dementia, what would *he* tell us?"
- Surrogates should work to respect the autonomous preferences of the patient.
- Autonomy exists only in the context of accurate physiologic parameters.
- An interdisciplinary team of medical specialists from different professions can help with optimal decision-making.

References

1. Mahon MM. An advance directive in two questions. *J Pain Symptom Manage.* 2011;41(4):801–807. doi:10.1016/j.jpainsymman.2011.01.002
2. Mahon MM. Advanced care decision making: Asking the right people the right questions. *J Psychosoc Nurs Ment Health Serv.* 2010;48(7):13–19. doi:10.3928/02793695-20100528-01
3. Appelbaum PS, Trachsel M. The doctrine of informed consent doesn't need modification for supported decision making. *Am J Bioeth.* 2021;21(11):27–29. doi:10.1080/15265161.2021.1980143
4. Torke AM, Alexander GC, Lantos J. Substituted judgment: The limitations of autonomy in surrogate decision making. *J Gen Intern Med.* 2008;23(9):1514-1517. doi:10.1007/s11606-008-0688-8
5. Peterson A, Karlawish J, Largent E. Supported decision making with people at the margins of autonomy. *Am J Bioethics.* 2021;21(11), 4–18. doi:10.1080/15265161.2020.1863507
6. Geddis-Regan A, Errington L, Abley C, Wassall R, Exley C, Thomson R. Enhancing shared and surrogate decision making for people living with dementia: A systematic review of the effectiveness of interventions. *Health Expect.* 2021;24(1):19–32. doi:10.1111/hex.13167

7. Ioannidis I, Ismael AM, Forssten MP, et al. The mortality burden in patients with hip fractures and dementia. *Eur J Trauma Emerg Surg.* 2022;48:2919–2925. https://doi.org/10.1007/s00068-021-01612-4

8. Sullivan NM, Blake LE, George M, Mears SC. Palliative care in the hip fracture patient. *Geriatr Orthop Surg Rehabil.* 2019;10. doi:10.1177/2151459319849801

9. van der Zwaard C, Stein CE, Bootsma JEM, van Geffen HJAA, Douw CM, Keijsers, CJPW. Fewer patients undergo surgery when adding a comprehensive geriatric assessment in older patients with a hip fracture. *Arch Orthop Trauma Surg.* 2019;140:487–492.

10. Hou M, Zhang Y, Chen AC, et al. The effects of dementia on the prognosis and mortality of hip fracture surgery: A systematic review and meta-analysis. *Aging Clin Exp Res.* 2021;33:3161–3172. https://doi.org/10.1007/s40520-021-01864-5

11. Jorrisen RN, Inacio MC, Cations M, et al. Effect of dementia on outcomes after surgically treated hip fractures in older adults. *J Arthroplasty.* 2021;36(9):3181–3186. https://doi.org/10.1016/j.arth.2021.04.030

32 Approaching Palliative Sedation at the End of Life

Abigail Lebovitz and Tamara Vesel

Dr. Miller is a 42-year-old plastic surgeon who was diagnosed with amyotrophic lateral sclerosis (ALS) 6 months ago. He lives in Massachusetts with his wife and two school-aged children. He has declined life-prolonging measures and is currently receiving hospice care. You and the hospice physician are consulted at the patient's request to meet with Dr. Miller and his family to discuss his goals of care. In your first meeting, Dr. Miller openly shares how his life has changed since his diagnosis with ALS. He describes the progressive symptoms that are negatively affecting his daily life. These include choking on food, being dependent on others for his care, and being bedridden. You feel this was a positive first encounter and laid the foundation to better understand and achieve his goals of care in the coming sessions. As the conversation is wrapping up, Dr. Miller requests, "I want to die after my wife's birthday in 2 months. Can you help me?" He is asking for physician-assisted dying.

What do you do now?

DISCUSSION

> The alleviation of suffering is an essential goal of medical care. To treat it, however, providers must first recognize pain and suffering.
>
> —Eric J. Cassell[1(p531)]

When approaching the end of life, many individuals are uninformed about the available care options. Different palliative measures are available to patients depending on the stage of illness and symptom experience. Early discussion of disease progression with patients with terminal illnesses and informed planning with patients and their families are critical components of providing high-quality medical care. As patients approach death, the goal of medicine is to improve quality of life and to decrease suffering and illness burden.

Our understanding of human suffering is complex. The best we understand suffering from a medical point of view is that suffering can be physical (including pain), psychological, existential, and spiritual. For most of the symptoms, we have the tools, pharmacological and nonpharmacological, to modify a patient's experience. Although symptoms may not be eliminated, they are typically reduced to adequately alleviate the suffering of the patient and family. However, we still encounter many patients approaching the end of life who are unable to find relief from their suffering; this experience is known as intolerable suffering. Despite intensified treatment efforts, the symptoms these patients continue to experience become refractory. Studies have demonstrated that delirium, dyspnea, severe pain, severe distress, and insomnia are the most common refractory symptoms cited in the initiation of palliative sedation (Table 32.1).[2,3] Because the experience of suffering is contingent on having a consciousness, these symptoms can be alleviated by decreasing an individual's consciousness. Without consciousness, humans do not suffer. In extreme situations, some patients are willing to let go of consciousness at the end of life with the goal of relieving their suffering.

When comfort is the principal care goal for a patient at the end of life, palliative sedation is a treatment tool that provides relief for extreme suffering that has been unrelieved by other aggressive treatment measures. Palliative sedation provides comfort and symptom relief at the end of life to patients with a prognosis of hours to days using sedation proportional

TABLE 32.1 Sample of Medications Used in Palliative Sedation

Drug Classification	Drug Name (Brand Name)	Dosing[a]
Benzodiazepines	Midazolam (Versed)	Loading dose: 0.03–0.05 mg/kg intravenous push over 5 min; repeat q5min until desired effect Continuous infusion: 0.02–0.1 mg/kg/hr; titrate to response
Barbiturates	Phenobarbital (Luminal)	Loading dose: 7.5 mg/kg × 1 over 1 hr Daily dose: 100–400 mg/day (divided q6h)
	Pentobarbital (Nembutal)	Loading dose: 10–15 mg/kg Continuous infusion: 1–4 mg/kg/hr
Short-acting anesthetics	Propofol (Diprivan)	Induction: Slow intravenous infusion of 100–150 µg/kg/min for 3–5 min or slow injection of 0.5 mg/kg over 3–5 min Maintenance: 15–65 µg/kg/min
Opioids[b]	Fentanyl	25–100 µg/hr continuous infusion
	Morphine	1–5 mg/hr continuous infusion
	Hydromorphone (Dilaudid)	0.2–1 mg/hr continuous infusion

[a]Dose ranges should be titrated to patients' sedative needs and may require dose adjustments that are outside of the ranges listed based on patient response.
[b]Opioid starting dose should be determined based on the patient's current pain regimen. If the patient is currently on opioids, start to titrate from current dosing, not on dosing recommendations for opiate naive patients.

to the patient's symptoms. The intent is to relieve severe distress, not to hasten death. It is not equal to voluntary active euthanasia or physician-assisted dying.

There is legal and professional support for the practice of palliative sedation in medicine in the United States and beyond when caring for an imminently dying patient with refractory symptoms.[4–7] The principle of double effect provides an ethical justification for palliative sedation.[8] This principle is used to explain the permissibility of an action that may cause a serious harm, such as death, as a side effect of bringing about a good end with overriding moral importance. When applying the principle of double effect, it must be impossible to bring about the good end without the harm.

Palliative sedation should only be implemented when all therapies have been considered, utilized, or failed. Standard therapies attempted and/or considered prior to palliative sedation may include, but are not limited to, medications (opioids, neuroleptics, anticonvulsants, anxiolytics, or antidepressants), neuromodulatory procedures (nerve blocks and intrathecal analgesia), palliative radiation therapies, and palliative surgical procedures. Prior to the initiation of palliative sedation, an active decision must be made to withhold life-sustaining measures including chest compressions, defibrillation, endotracheal intubation, mechanical ventilation, and cardiovascular support. If there is an implanted defibrillator, it must be deactivated. Under most circumstances, the routine use of vital sign monitoring should be minimized or stopped for comfort.[9] Medications that are used for palliative sedation in patients with refractory symptoms at the end of life include benzodiazepines, first-generation antipsychotics, barbiturates, and short-acting anesthetics (Table 32.2).

The utilization of palliative sedation is highly variable worldwide. National and international guidelines exist,[4] and variability is most likely attributed to physician knowledge and what is labeled palliative sedation in clinical practice. Many studies have attempted to measure the impact of palliative sedation on patient survival, and the overall conclusion is that survival is the same (or even longer) when sedated patients are compared with nonsedated patients.[3,10,11] Palliative sedation is distinct from voluntary active euthanasia. Voluntary active euthanasia is a deliberate termination of life by active intervention, usually at the request

TABLE 32.2 **Examples of Reasons for Initiation of Palliative Sedation**

Physical	Psychological	Existential	Spiritual
Refractory pain	Delirium	Existential suffering	Spiritual suffering
Dyspnea	Agitation		
Emesis	Uncontrolled anxiety		
Nausea			
Intractable seizures			

of the patient. Physician-assisted dying is similar to voluntary active euthanasia in that death is the intended consequence, but the patient self-administers the medication. By contrast, the intent of palliative sedation is relief from refractory symptoms, not expressly to end the life of the suffering patient; death of the patient is not a criterion used to gauge success of the treatment. As of 2022, in the United States, legalization of physician-assisted dying was regulated at the state level, and voluntary active euthanasia was not permitted anywhere. Worldwide, the legalization of physician-assisted dying and voluntary active euthanasia is constantly evolving. Data from the Netherlands, the first European nation to legalize euthanasia in 2001, show euthanasia accounted for 4.5% of total deaths in 2021.[12]

It is the role of clinicians to identify individuals with terminal illnesses who are likely to benefit from palliative sedation. The decision to use palliative sedation should be based on an informed, collaborative decision-making process with a multidisciplinary care team, the patient, and the patient's family or health care proxy. When considering palliative sedation, clear communication by the care team to the patient and the patient's family and health care proxy is integral. When the decision of palliative sedation is made through collaborative decision-making and comprehensive informed consent, detailed documentation by the attending physician is required. Planning and implementation of palliative sedation require a trusted relationship between the physician, other health care providers, the patient, and the patient's family.

As a clinician, what do you do when your patient asks you to help them die? How do you respond to a person who is asking you something that may be unprofessional or even illegal? The human impulse can be to rush to judgment, often reminding the patient of the illegitimacy of the request. We do not want to devalue the patient due to our discomfort or inexperience. It is the clinician's responsibility to have knowledge of what is legal and not legal, doable and not doable. You may have negative personal feelings, but you should make the best effort to engage as impartially as possible and explore the extent of a patient's experience that led to the request. As the clinician, you may further probe the root cause of the suffering by asking, "Tell me more, what symptoms are you experiencing that may be causing you to ask me this? What keeps you awake at night?" or "Giving up on life is a serious request. Tell me more about what you are experiencing now or worrying about in the future that is making you ask for this request?"

As a clinician, one must be able to hear and to process with patients their requests about dying. This can be a difficult task, and all clinicians should recognize their discomfort with these requests. Clinicians have an obligation to accept someone's experience of suffering as valid. It is the role of a clinician to explore the patient's experience from multiple angles and to work to understand why the patient's life has lost its value. As one approaches the topic of suffering, particularly beyond the point of physical pain, the clinician and patient enter an intimate space beyond our usual encounters in medicine. These difficult encounters and decision-making processes highlight the need to lead with empathy and compassion when approaching palliative sedation and end-of-life care.

CASE RESOLUTION

From his initial request, Dr. Miller and his physician team dive into a conversation about care options, ethical and legal considerations, and patient-specific goals and concerns about the end of life. Given that Dr. Miller lives in Massachusetts, physician-assisted dying is not currently a legal option for his care.

Over time, the physician discovers that Dr. Miller fears choking on his own saliva, a common fear and symptom in individuals suffering with ALS. As a surgeon, he has watched patients waking up from anesthesia choking after surgery, and, for him, this is an unacceptable way of dying. He fears dying of respiratory distress and does not want to prolong his family's suffering while he is dying. His physician counsels Dr. Miller on how they can approach his fears, and they discuss what is permissible. They will first try to manage his symptoms through supportive measures. If they can no longer do so and he is suffering from respiratory distress, they will consider using palliative sedation to treat his refractory symptoms. Extensive education around palliative sedation is provided to the patient and his family. Although he had once considered suicide, Dr. Miller realizes that palliative sedation is the most appropriate option for himself and his family.

The birthday of his wife arrives, and Dr. Miller does not ask to die. He is having more difficulty swallowing his own saliva, but he has not had any symptomatic aspiration episodes. As time passes, he no longer wants to die on this day. Instead, he will wait until specific symptoms occur. He finds comfort in having a clear plan with his physician team. Dr. Miller begins dictating a memoir as a keepsake for his children and family; his narrative changes to what he can keep behind as a legacy.

Months pass by and Dr. Miller's health declines. He calls the physician and asks for intravenous hydration; although this is not a traditional treatment at the end of life, he wants to see how he will respond. A week later, his wife calls and says it is time—Dr. Miller is choking and can no longer tolerate his increased respiratory distress. Prior to initiating palliative sedation, his physician is present as Dr. Miller says his final good-bye to his family and friends. His priest engages the group in spiritual prayer. Dr. Miller is sedated to a level of unconsciousness and is cared for by his family, friends, and the hospice team until he dies 9 days later.

KEY POINTS TO REMEMBER

- People with life-threatening illness/end-stage disease may suffer from severe symptoms that are not ameliorated by usual medical and palliative interventions.
- When the overriding goal is comfort for the person, palliative sedation provides a means to relieve extreme suffering.
- Refractory symptoms include physical, psychological, spiritual, and existential symptoms.
- Palliative sedation is distinct from voluntary active euthanasia and physician-assisted dying; palliative sedation does not hasten death.
- Clinician empathy and openness to the exploration of patients' experiences and expectations with suffering are critical to approach the decision to plan for and to initiate palliative sedation at the end of life.

References

1. Cassell EJ. Diagnosing suffering: A perspective. *Ann Intern Med.* 1999;131(7):531–534. doi:10.7326/0003-4819-131-7-199910050-00009

2. Chiu TY, Hu WY, Lue BH, Cheng SY, Chen CY. Sedation for refractory symptoms of terminal cancer patients in Taiwan. *J Pain Symptom Manage.* 2001;21(6):467–472. doi:10.1016/s0885-3924(01)00286-x

3. Schur S, Weixler D, Gabl C, et al. Sedation at the end of life: A nation-wide study in palliative care units in Austria. *BMC Palliat Care.* 2016;15:50. doi:10.1186/s12904-016-0121-8

4. Abarshi E, Rietjens J, Robijn L, et al. International variations in clinical practice guidelines for palliative sedation: A systematic review [Published correction appears in *BMJ Support Palliat Care.* 2018 Jun;8(2):239]. *BMJ Support Palliat Care.* 2017;7(3):223–229. doi:10.1136/bmjspcare-2016-001159

5. American Academy of Hospice and Palliative Medicine. Statement on palliative sedation. 2016. http://aahpm.org/positions/palliative-sedation

6. Cherny NI, Radbruch L; Board of the European Association for Palliative Care. European Association for Palliative Care (EAPC) recommended framework for the use of sedation in palliative care. *Palliat Med.* 2009;23(7):581–593. doi:10.1177/0269216309107024

7. HPNA Position Paper: Palliative sedation at the end of life. *J Hosp Palliat Nurs.* 2003;5(4):235–237. https://journals.lww.com/jhpn/Fulltext/2003/10000/HPNA_Position_Paper__Palliative_Sedation_at_the.22.aspx

8. McIntyre A. Doctrine of double effect. In: *Stanford Encyclopedia of Philosophy* (Spring 2019 edition). Published December 24, 2018. Accessed December 20, 2022. https://plato.stanford.edu/entries/double-effect

9. Cherny NI; ESMO Guidelines Working Group. ESMO clinical practice guidelines for the management of refractory symptoms at the end of life and the use of palliative sedation. *Ann Oncol.* 2014;25(Suppl 3):iii143–iii152. doi:10.1093/annonc/mdu238

10. Beller EM, van Driel ML, McGregor L, Truong S, Mitchell G. Palliative pharmacological sedation for terminally ill adults. *Cochrane Database Syst Rev.* 2015;1(1):CD010206. doi:10.1002/14651858.CD010206.pub2

11. Maeda I, Morita T, Yamaguchi T, et al. Effect of continuous deep sedation on survival in patients with advanced cancer (J-Proval): A propensity score-weighted analysis of a prospective cohort study. *Lancet Oncol.* 2016;17(1):115–122. doi:10.1016/S1470-2045(15)00401-5

12. Netherlands Regional Euthanasia Review Committees. Home page. 2022. https://english.euthanasiecommissie.nl

Further Reading

Arevalo JJ, Rietjens JA, Swart SJ, Perez RS, van der Heide A. Day-to-day care in palliative sedation: Survey of nurses' experiences with decision-making and performance. *Int J Nurs Stud.* 2013;50(5):613–621. doi:10.1016/j.ijnurstu.2012.10.004

Cherny NI, on behalf of ESMO Guidelines Working Group. ESMO clinical practice guidelines for the management of refractory symptoms at the end of life and the use of palliative sedation. *Ann Oncol.* 2014;25(Suppl 3):143–152. doi:10.1093/annonc/mdu238

Maltoni M, Setola E. Palliative sedation in patients with cancer. *Cancer Control.* 2015;22(4):433–441. doi:10.1177/107327481502200409

33 Advance Care Planning

Nnamdi C. Iwuala and Lauren Shaiova

Mr. Brown has widely metastatic prostate cancer. He is concerned that his son may prevent the medical team from following his wishes. He is asking what documents can be put in place to have his wishes followed at the end of life (advance directives and durable power of attorney).

What do you do now?

DISCUSSION

Patients with advanced cancer confront significant life changes as they adapt to living with serious illness, negotiate frequent medical encounters, cope with symptoms, and face death.[1] This group commonly has concerns about the dying process, loss of control, and dignity. The desire to control one's health care decisions is a core construct codified by the bioethical principles of autonomy and the right to self-determination.[2]

Medical and legal provisions exist that ensure patients receive future medical care, especially end-of-life care, consistent with their values, goals, and preferences. The process of delineating, documenting, and implementing an individual's future medical and end-of-life care choices has evolved from a purely legal approach to the favored communicative approach, called advance care planning (ACP). ACP is a process in which patients, their families or other chosen decision-makers, and their health care providers reflect on the patients' goals, values, and beliefs; discuss how they should inform current and future medical care; and ultimately use this information to document the patients' future health choices accurately.[3]

Advance directives (ADs) are essential tools that result from the process of ACP and convey a patient's future health choices. There are many types of ADs; the most recognized are the living will and durable power of attorney for health care. The living will is a legal document that states an individual's specific health care preferences for life-sustaining treatments and resuscitation. The durable power of attorney is a signed legal document that appoints a surrogate decision-maker (also known as health care agent or proxy) to make medical decisions on the patient's behalf if the patient loses decisional capacity. A major limitation of the living will is that although it is a legally valid expression of a patient's wishes, doctors and paramedic staff are not legally required to adhere to it even when it is accessible. As such, they give no legal guarantee that a patient will not receive unwanted care, such as resuscitation and intubation, in an emergency.

To address these limitations, the Physician Orders for Life-Sustaining Treatment (POLST) paradigm was created in Oregon in 1991. POLST (known as Medical Orders for Life-Sustaining Treatment [MOLST] in some states) is an approach to ACP used for patients with advanced cancer and other advanced life-limiting medical conditions or advanced frailty to delineate and document their here-and-now goals for medical decisions that could confront the patients in the immediate future.[4] When signed by a patient (or their surrogate) and the physician, the POLST document is both a medical order and a legal document that is respected and followed by paramedic staff and physicians across all care settings and scenarios. AD and POLST tools are complimentary and aim to cover all situations and scenarios that people with advanced cancer and other advanced life-limiting illnesses may face (Table 33.1).

TABLE 33.1   **Differences Between POLST and Advance Directives**

	POLST Form	Advance Directives
Type of document?	Medical order	Legal document
Who completes?	Health care professional (who can sign varies by state: https://polst.org/state-signature-requirements-pdf)	Individual
Who needs one?	Any patients considered to be at risk for a life-threatening clinical event because they have a serious life-limiting medical condition, which may include advanced frailty	All competent adults
Is completion voluntary?	Yes	Yes
Appoints a surrogate?	No	Yes
Can patient's surrogate complete, change, or void?	In most states, yes	No
What is communicated?	Specific medical orders	General wishes about treatment wishes

Continued

TABLE 33.1 **Continued**

	POLST Form	Advance Directives
Can emergency personnel follow?	Yes	No
Ease in locating?	Should be easy. Patient has original. Copy is in medical record. Copy may be in a registry (if state has a registry).	May be difficult. Depends on where individual keeps it and if they have told someone where it is, given a copy to surrogate, or to health care professional to put in their medical record.
Periodic review?	Health care professional is responsible for reviewing with patient or surrogate upon transfer to a new facility; when there is a substantial change in patient's medical condition; or when patient's goals of care or treatment preferences change.	Up to the individual about how often it is reviewed and/or updated.

POLST, Physician Orders for Life-Sustaining Treatment.
Adapted from the National POLST Coalition (https://polst.org/wp-content/uploads/2020/06/2020.06.05-Chart-Comparing-Advance-Directives-and-POLST.pdf).

Aligning the care that patients receive at the end of life with their wishes entails several actions and steps. A crucial step is the appointment of a surrogate (also called a health care proxy or agent) using the durable power of attorney for health care. The surrogate acts as the patient's health care decision-maker if the patient loses decisional capacity. It is imperative that the patient chooses a surrogate who knows them well, understands their values and choices, would advocate for them, and whom they trust to carry out their wishes. It is also important to have an ACP consultation with their medical provider to discuss their current health problems, prognosis, future medical decisions that may arise, and their preferences and care goals. Portable medical orders (POLST), respected across various care settings, including the patient's home, can be created during these patient–health care provider encounters.

Family members are most often named surrogates. However, the complexity and emotional stress involved in making end-of-life decisions for family members sometimes cause conflict between the patient's wishes and the family member's desires, which may lead to end-of-life care that deviates from the patient's wishes. Such family conflicts inform the choice of non-family members as a surrogate by some patients. Although family members cannot overrule legally appointed surrogates without resorting to judicial proceedings, patients are encouraged to involve their family in the advance care planning discussions to reduce the likelihood of family opposition.

CASE RESOLUTION

Mr. Brown's concern that his son may prevent his medical team from following his wishes reflects the concern for loss of control and health care autonomy, common among people with advanced life-limiting illnesses.

The first step in ensuring Mr. Brown gets the end-of-life care consistent with his values and goals is that he starts the process of advance care planning while he still has decisional capacity. Deep reflection about his values, preferences, and goals and his idea of a good death is necessary. Meeting with his health care provider to discuss his clinical condition, preferences for care, and medical decisional challenges ahead is recommended. His surrogate should accompany him to the visit with his health care provider, if possible.

Communicating his preferences and goals with his chosen surrogate through multiple discussions enables the surrogate to have a well-rounded understanding of his wishes and to make decisions concordant with it. Mr. Brown should also make these preferences known to his son and family members to reduce conflict when the time comes for implementation. After completing his AD documents (living will and durable power of attorney for health care, which names his surrogate), he should store them safely and give copies to his surrogate and medical care provider.

Due to Mr. Brown's advanced cancer and his proximity to the end of his life, it is imperative that his medical provider completes a POLST form based on Mr. Brown's expressed wishes and incorporates a copy of the document in his medical records. Mr. Brown should keep the original POLST in a visible area in his residence and take it with him when visiting a health care facility.

With the appointment of a surrogate and creation of a POLST document signed by his physician, Mr. Brown's wishes, preferences, and goals for end-of-life care are made clear and actionable across various care settings or care levels and his concerns addressed.

KEY POINTS TO REMEMBER

- Patient autonomy and the right to self-determination are essential tenets of modern health care.
- ACP is a comprehensive process that delineates, documents, and facilitates implementation of future medical and end-of-life care goals.
- Living wills have the limitation that health care providers are not required or bound to adhere to them.
- Durable power of attorney for health care can be used to appoint a legally empowered health care surrogate or proxy, a crucial component of ACP.
- Portable medical orders (POLST) are legally binding medical orders applicable across various health care settings and the patient's home.

References

1. Rodenbach RA, Althouse AD, Schenker Y, et al. Relationships between advanced cancer patients' worry about dying and illness understanding, treatment preferences, and advance care planning. *J Pain Symptom Manage.* 2021;61(4):723–731. doi:10.1016/j.jpainsymman.2020.09.004

2. Volker DL, Wu HL. Cancer patients' preferences for control at the end of life. *Qual Health Res.* 2011;21(12):1618–1631. doi:10.1177/1049732311415287

3. Silveira MJ. Advance care planning and advance directives. UpToDate. n.d. Accessed February 22, 2023. https://www.uptodate.com/contents/advance-care-planning-and-advance-directives
4. National POLST Coalition. POLST: Portable medical orders for seriously ill or frail individuals. 2022. Accessed February 25, 2023. https://polst.org

Further Reading

Quill TE. *Primer of Palliative Care*. 7th ed. American Academy of Hospice and Palliative Medicine; 2019.

34 Substituted Judgment

Gabriel Lutz

John and Dave own a home and have lived together for 30 years. They are retired and share finances, although they have never legally married. One morning while home alone, Dave experiences sudden vision loss, muscle weakness, and loss of consciousness. Several hours later, John returns home to find Dave unresponsive on the floor. Dave is admitted to the local hospital and found with a large ischemic stroke. John is at the bedside when Dave's parents arrive to find their son unresponsive and connected to numerous artificial life-support systems. Dave's consultant neurologist shares that his chances for a meaningful neurologic recovery are near zero and asks what Dave's wishes would be regarding long-term artificial support.

John recalls a recent conversation in which Dave, having recently witnessed a close friend become severely ill, adamantly expressed not wanting to be kept alive indefinitely on life-support if he could not return to his previous quality of life. After John shares this information, Dave's parents exclaim, "Don't listen to John, he and Dave aren't even married! Please, do everything you can to keep our son alive!"

What do you do now?

DISCUSSION

In this scenario, we are faced with two ethical challenges. First is the challenge of identifying the treatment wishes of an incapacitated person. An *advance directive*, completed while a patient retains capacity, is the best tool with which to identify an individual's core values that can guide their wishes for treatment. Although laws vary between states, most will do their best to respect wishes designated in an advance directive even if completed out of state. In the absence of an advance directive, *substituted judgment* must be used to identify the decisions an individual would make for themself—that is, to identify what choices a reasonable individual would make to best serve their interests, such as pursuing renewal of health when possible or avoidance of pain and suffering when possible.[1]

The second challenge is finding the person(s) best suited to exercise substituted judgment in order to guide care for patients—known as identifying a medical decision-maker.[2] This issue arises commonly regardless of the location or specialty you practice. Identifying the correct person(s) for making health care decisions may sometimes be very challenging. Some individuals may be unfit to make their own treatment choices because they are unable to fully comprehend the severity of their illness, but they may still retain the ability to name an adult they trust to make medical decisions on their behalf; this person is known as a *health care agent*. If an agent agrees to serve in this role, their authority in decision-making supersedes all others.[3] An individual can choose to name nearly anyone they wish to be their agent, and the person need not be directly related; however, an agent cannot be an employee of the health care facility in which an individual is receiving care.

If no agent exists, then the surrogacy hierarchy comes into effect. The hierarchy designates individuals as surrogate medical decision-makers depending on their level of presumed familiarity with a patient. If nobody is available from a given class, the search continues in the next class of lower hierarchy. For example, a patient's spouse or domestic partner is the first surrogate; if no such person is available, then all adult children (equally) are consulted next, followed by parents, then all adult siblings (equally), and finally a friend who is familiar enough to know a patient's wishes. A surrogate may only consent to withdrawal of life-sustaining medical treatment if appropriate medical staff determine a patient to be in a persistent vegetative state or in a terminal/end-stage condition.[3]

Briefly, a domestic partnership is a relationship in which two unmarried, unrelated adults, *regardless of gender*, are mutually dependent on each other for their personal, financial, and domestic well-being (potentially including shared joint responsibility in child-rearing). The specific duration of a relationship was (but no longer is) a part of the definition of domestic partnership.

Even after identifying the appropriate individuals, it is not uncommon to find surrogates of equal hierarchy disagreeing. In such cases, holding a family meeting is the best initial step toward the goal of arriving at a unified decision. Any given individual has the right to forfeit only their own decision-making privilege, leaving the task to others of the same hierarchy. If a shared decision cannot be achieved, the prudent next step is to contact an ethics consultant.

Occasionally, an individual may be deemed legally incompetent due to some form of disability. These vulnerable individuals may receive a court-appointed guardian to aid with personal/medical or financial needs depending on their specific disability. Although less common, this scenario is important for providers to be aware of, specifically whether legal guardians have been granted medical decision-making rights; in such cases, guardians are the prevailing medical decision-makers tasked with deciding which treatments are in the patient's best interests.

CASE RESOLUTION

As the primary physician, you recommend a family meeting with Dave's parents and domestic partner John. Although initially tense, both parties begin cooperating as they realize they all love Dave dearly and strive to do their best to respect his wishes. Dave's parents recognize that their initial request was incongruent with who they knew their son to be, and they accept that he would not want to continue living in his current debilitated condition. You confirm no prior advance directive nor health care power of attorney forms have been completed, leaving John as the primary surrogate medical decision-maker. John requests for Dave to be compassionately withdrawn from artificial life support machines. Surrounded by his partner and parents, Dave dies peacefully later that afternoon.

KEY POINTS TO REMEMBER

- A health care surrogate should be aware they are being asked to employ substituted judgment in their decision-making—that is, to decide as they believe the patient would, not what the surrogate would choose for themself in such a situation.
- In terms of decision-making hierarchy, first would be an agent named by the patient (or a guardian if court appointed). Next would be a spouse/domestic partner, adult children, parents, siblings, and significant friend/other relative.
- In order to qualify as a domestic partner, an individual must live with the patient and share significant finances. Neither gender nor a predetermined period of time is considered.
- Consider an ethics consultation if there is disagreement on who should serve as a patient's surrogate(s) or if there is significant disagreement between decision-makers.

References
1. Macauley RC. *Ethics in Palliative Care*. Oxford University Press; 2018:61–70.
2. Jaworska A. Advance directives and substitute decision-making. In: *Stanford Encyclopedia of Philosophy*. Published March 24, 2009. Accessed November 23, 2023. https://plato.stanford.edu/entries/advance-directives
3. Maryland Office of the Attorney General. Health Care Decisions Act: Text and educational materials. n.d. Accessed November 18, 2023. https://www.maryland attorneygeneral.gov/Pages/HealthPolicy/hcda.aspx

Further Reading
Acquaviva K. *LGBTQ-Inclusive Hospice and Palliative Care: A Practical Guide to Transforming Professional Practice*. Harrington Park Press; 2017.